Arthritis and Back Pain: Exercises for the Bath

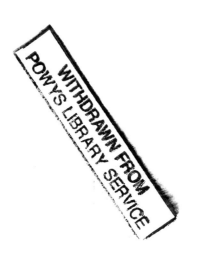

JUDY JETTER and NANCY KADLEC

ARTHRITIS
— AND —
BACK PAIN:
EXERCISES
— FOR —
THE BATH

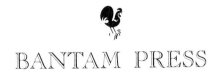

BANTAM PRESS

LONDON · NEW YORK · TORONTO · SYDNEY · AUCKLAND

TRANSWORLD PUBLISHERS LTD
61-63 Uxbridge Road, London W5 5SA

TRANSWORLD PUBLISHERS (AUSTRALIA) PTY LTD
15-23 Helles Avenue, Moorebank NSW 2170, Australia

TRANSWORLD PUBLISHERS (NZ) LTD
Cnr Moselle and Waipareira Aves,
Henderson, Auckland

Published 1987 by Bantam Press,
a division of Transworld Publishers Ltd
Copyright © Judy Jetter and Nancy Kedlec 1986

British Library Cataloguing in Publication Data

Jetter, Judy
    Arthritis & backpain : exercises for the bath.
    1. Backache—Treatment   2. Hydrotherapy
    I. Title II. Kadlec, Nancy
    616.7'220653   RD768

    ISBN 0-593-01274-7

Printed and bound in Great Britain by
Biddles Ltd, Guildford and King's Lynn

For Bill, with love

Contents

Special thanks to the Chicagoland Spine Center and to the National Arthritis Foundation for their excellent work in the fields of both education and practical application of methods to reduce or relieve chronic pain.

Arthritis and Back Pain: Exercises for the Bath

Introduction

Arthritis and back pain in their many and varied forms are the two most prevalent disabling medical conditions of modern society. Back pain can result from a wide variety of causes including, but certainly not limited to, arthritis itself. Self-diagnosis is both foolish and dangerous. A doctor should be consulted whenever pain persists or is severe. After diagnosis medical treatment often includes exercise therapy for the back itself, as well as to strengthen the abdominal muscles, which should take the brunt of the load from the shorter and weaker muscles of the back.

Doctors have long recognized the benefits of exercise as an important part of health care. That is why they frequently recommend a comprehensive programme of exercise as an adjunct to medication or other forms of treatment for the total health care of their patients who suffer from arthritis or back pain. Physical- and occupational-therapy programmes are routinely ordered, generally within the hospital setting. Unfortunately, these programmes are usually discontinued once a patient is released and are seldom restarted unless the patient is hospitalized again. Doctors who recommend that a patient exercise, often specifically in water, usually give no specific guidelines to the actual exercises themselves. Part of the problem is that until now it has been difficult to find a book of aquatic exercises written and illustrated for the layman.

All the exercises in this book have been selected and approved by Nancy Kadlec, a registered occupational therapist with more than twenty years of experience in both hospital and private settings. The text was written by Judy Jetter, a former aquatic-exercise and swimming instructor. Judy and Nancy, along with Judy's husband, Bill, demonstrate all the exercises in the photographs throughout this book. Judy and Bill's son, Steve Sheehy, appears in several photographs in the spa section.

All the exercises have been designed to be done in your own home. Most can be done in a standard bathtub, although those involving side-to-side movements are more easily and more efficiently done in certain types of spas or hot tubs that allow for a wider range of movement. If you decide to use a public facility, it should be checked for temperature and compliance with common-sense safety procedures such as adequate use of chemical disinfectants, convenient hand-rails, and non-skid walkways and stairs. All of the exercises can be done in a spa, no matter in which section they appear, even though they may be illustrated in a bathtub.

Our exercises should become an integral part of your home health-care regimen. They develop strength, flexibility and co-ordination, gently and safely, in joints affected by arthritis, back pain, and even stroke or pain and paralysis resulting from accidental trauma or other damage, and provide a fuller range of joint movement for anyone performing them on a regular basis. Because they are geared to any level of strength and endurance, you will gradually be able to increase your stamina. They should never be done so vigorously that pain results.

People who begin their exercise programme in a severely weakened condition are urged to perform only two or three repetitions of each exercise that they are able to do and skip the ones that are too difficult initially. As pain and stiffness decrease, the exercises can be done more quickly and with more repetitions of the same exercise. The time certain positions are held can also increase from a slow count of three to a maximum of twelve, where each count corresponds to roughly one second. To increase flexibility and strength further, mass and drag can be added in the form of clothing and wrist- and ankle-weights, if your doctor approves. Even when your muscles and joints are only minimally stiff and sore, you will still get a great deal of benefit from the soothing warmth of the heated water combined with medically sound principles of range of motion and strengthening.

These exercises can be performed in conjunction with *The Arthritis Book of Water Exercise*, in which we outlined a series of exercises primarily suitable for pool, lake or ocean, but which also contains a chapter on home exercises.

One final word about illness is in order before proceeding to the next chapter. Many people are tempted to self-diagnose recurring aches and pains as arthritis or some sort of non-specific, transient muscle strain in the back, and to self-prescribe popular exercise programmes or medication from the myriad of over-the-counter compounds available at any chemist's shop. To do so is extremely foolish. Long-term use of any drugs can be safely prescribed only by a qualified doctor who can simultaneously evaluate the desirability of exercise therapy. Certain very serious diseases show symptoms very similar to arthritis or to simple back strain. You can cause yourself serious permanent harm by relying on self-diagnosis and any self-administered medication or exercise regimen as a substitute for thorough, comprehensive medical diagnosis and treatment for recurring pain.

1

The Myth of the Magic Bullet

Desperate people sometimes fool themselves for a time into believing that there is a simple cure for the arthritis or for the severe chronic back pain that plagues their lives, if only they can find it. They are mistaken. Just as chronic back pain often requires a permanent change in life-style together with some fairly complex medical procedures, sometimes including surgery, the pain and potentially physically disabling body changes of arthritis have not yet yielded to a simple medical cure. In fact, no cure for arthritis has yet been developed, nor has any of the extensive research into this potentially debilitating disease promised the hope of a cure in the foreseeable future. No matter what claims are made for a product, book, diet programme or exercise regimen, it must be remembered that, although the symptoms of arthritis can sometimes be controlled by the judicious use of medication combined with medically sound exercises that maintain or build flexibility and strength, the disease itself is incurable. One reason no one has yet found a remedy is that the disease presents itself in so many forms.

More than a hundred different types of arthritis have been recognized and diagnosed. Arthritis affects every age group from infants to the elderly. There is little doubt, however, that the percentage of older people who are afflicted with some form of this disease is much higher than that of the rest of the general population. This is in part because of the normal wear and tear of the ageing process on the joints.

Back problems, on the other hand, are most prevalent in young men, although either sex can experience chronic back pain at any age. It can often be cured, but the path to recovery can take many different turns. Sometimes just eliminating certain tasks or movements can bring relief. At other times bed rest is recommended. Surgery is the last resort, but new techniques including enzyme injections have made curing certain types of back pain safer and more comfortable for the patient. No matter what the patient's age, however, back pain often recurs unless and until some permanent life-style changes are made. Often these involve simple common sense coupled with an exercise regimen.

Any exercise programme undertaken by a person with arthritis or back pain should have a doctor's approval and must be done with specific precautions in mind. For example, moving any part of your body past the point where comfort ends and severe discomfort or outright pain results is *not* recommended unless your doctor specifically advises you to do so. Despite the fact that the popular 'No pain, no gain' philosophy of exercise touted by some healthy but medically uninformed Hollywood stars, marathon-runners, and many exercise instructors implies that pain is always good for you, nothing could be farther from the truth. Anyone who suffers from chronic pain cannot treat his or her body in the same manner as those who are pain-free. Pain-sufferers can damage their bodies permanently by overstressing joints. Even some instructors in nationally recognized exercise and fitness organizations may unknowingly be dispensing potentially harmful misinformation because their level of knowledge and academic training, although adequate for the healthy general public, is inadequate when dealing with chronic pain.

It is clear that today people are taking more responsibility for their own health maintenance rather than leaving health care entirely to a doctor, who in the past was expected to be an infallible source of magical pills or injections guaranteed to eliminate pain and potential disfigurement for ever. Such unrealistic reliance on doctors and drugs more often than not brought only frustration and loss of confidence in a doctor who, in many instances, was doing all that he could.

There are a number of medications for the treatment of arthritis. Each has a considerable range of effectiveness, as well as a broad range of side-effects, depending on the individual characteristics of the user. Simple non-prescription aspirin is generally recommended initially, but a person may progress to any of a multitude of highly advertised, highly priced prescription or non-prescription drugs, including steroids and metals such as gold. It is well to remember that none of these medications offers a cure for arthritis, no matter how slickly the advertisement is worded. Most do offer temporary relief from pain, at least to some degree. Some actually decrease swelling in red and painful immobile joints. Sometimes they can even help your body to boost its own natural counter-offensive against this disease, which can lead to a remission of symptoms lasting from several weeks to many years. In some cases the process by which they work is still not entirely clear.

Just as there is no 'magic bullet', there is no magic exercise regimen, no matter what the purveyors of phoney cures may claim. Regular exercise is important to your health, but it is only one of a number of interconnected factors that combine to contribute to balanced medical care. Your doctor is the mediator of that care and should tailor any programme to fit your individual health needs. For example, some people with arthritis or back pain also have severe hypertension, even though the two are not related. Of course, any number of other diseases can strike a person with arthritis – or he or she may be perfectly healthy otherwise. Don't take chances with your health. See your doctor and listen to the advice you are given. Then together you can work out a programme for your total physical well-being.

2

Getting Started

Water is the ideal exercise medium. It minimizes harmful gravitational effects of land-based exercises while strengthening muscles by its natural resistance, very much like today's hi-tech, highly touted, and expensive modern gym exercise equipment. Eighty-nine per cent of your body weight on land is suspended by the natural buoyancy of the water. Warm water also soothes aching, inflamed muscles.

Our primary goal is to help sufferers of chronic arthritis and back pain, but these exercises are equally valuable to anyone with muscle, joint or any other type of skeletal or tissue stiffness or tenderness, whether caused by an accident, surgery or some other condition. Stroke patients should pay particular attention to the passive-movement exercises in Chapter 5. They exercise paralysed limbs or muscles that are so weak they cannot move spontaneously.

Before beginning this programme of exercise, it is important that you know and follow some basic guidelines in order to maximize the benefits offered by the programme and to avoid possible pitfalls.

SAFETY PRECAUTIONS

Everyone knows that it is very dangerous to have electrical appliances such as radios or portable television sets near a bath tub where they can fall in. Bathtub exercisers must also be careful not to balance hair-driers or electric curling-tongs, electric shavers, clocks and so forth on a sink or window-ledge where they might accidentally be knocked into the water during exercise. *An appliance doesn't have to be turned on to be lethal. It just has to be plugged in.*

Bath rails are a must if you are unsteady on your feet. Wall-mounted grab-bars can also be placed behind and at the sides of hot tubs and spas. Installing and using them can help prevent dangerous falls, whether you are exercising or merely bathing.

Most newer bath tubs have built-in anti-skid strips, but you may still want some additional protection against slipping while getting into or out of the bath and while exercising. You must be sure that you can control the depth of your body in the water at all times, especially if you are small and your feet don't reach the end of the bath when you sit up. Do not rely on a bath towel to keep your body in place. Special non-skid strips, decals and rubber mats are available in most hardware stores.

It is always best to exercise or bathe when someone else is within calling distance. Never use soap or bath oil before you have finished exercising; they tend to make the bath slippery enough to cause an accident.

STARTING SLOWLY

Begin your exercise programme slowly, especially the first day or two. Gradually increase the number of repetitions of each exercise, as you build strength and endurance. Keep in mind your own capacity for each exercise and your doctor's advice about which exercises to stress – and which to eliminate. Nothing will be gained by exerting yourself to the point of pain or exhaustion on the first day, and then spending the next several days recuperating and dreading the thought of subsequent exercise sessions.

Avoid bouncing or other rapid, jerky movements that can harm tender swollen joints. Pay attention to special cautionary notes relating to specific exercises if you have the medical condition they describe. Otherwise, you may do your body more harm than good. People with arthritis must understand that the disease is often unpredictable. Exercises that are simple one day may be next to impossible twenty-four hours later. Listen to your body and be guided by what it tells you. If a joint screams enough, ease off and try again during the next session. The key to success is slow, steady progress over a sustained period of time.

Unless your doctor specifically tells you otherwise, go only as far as you can without pain when performing any of these exercises, no matter what range of movement is illustrated. Pain is nature's way of telling you to take it easy for your own good. Added flexibility may come with time and practice.

At the end of each exercise we have indicated the body areas affected, and we have summarized the exercises benefiting each area in our chart on pages 144-49. You need not be concerned if you don't feel movement or tension in the parts of your body listed for a particular exercise. Follow the instructions and illustrations as well as you can and you will obtain the maximum benefit for *your* body.

Your doctor may recommend that you modify some of these exercises, or omit one or more. Always listen to his or her recommendations. No one knows your medical needs better.

We do not recommend that you do any of these exercises on land. They are meant for water and can strain tender joints and muscles in a non-aquatic environment.

SOME TIPS ON TEMPERATURE AND WHEN TO EXERCISE

Water temperature should be comfortably warm to relax tight, sore muscles and joints, and should range somewhere between 85°F to a maximum of 90°F (30°C to 32°C), if you plan to exercise at a moderate to fast pace. The total time you spend in a heated tub or spa must be carefully monitored, and is dependent on the temperature of the water.

It is unwise to spend more than forty-five minutes exercising at elevated temperatures. If the temperature is between 91°F and 95°F (35°C), twenty minutes is enough. Time and effort spent exercising in water hotter than 99° (37°C) should

10

be minimal; a few gentle stretches and some passive and isometric exercises lasting several minutes are ample. Extremely hot water is debilitating and will put extra stress on your heart. Spa and hot tub manufacturers may recommend that water temperatures are safe even at 104°F or 105°F (about 40°C), but bear in mind that they are not recommending that you exercise in such superheated conditions, merely that you assume a relaxed, comfortable pose and soak your body. Don't increase the water temperature past 100°F (38°C) if you plan to exercise for more than a minute or two. Discontinue exercise immediately if you feel faint or nauseated.

People with high blood pressure or heart conditions are warned against prolonged bathing in water hotter than 99°F. It is best to check with your doctor before increasing the water temperature past this point. We recommend that you do not.

Under no circumstances should the aerobic portion of your programme be performed for longer than twenty minutes for the first several sessions, no matter what the water temperature. Most people will not be able to sustain even this amount of effort in the beginning. You may gradually increase the time you spend on the aerobic exercises, but we suggest that you lower the water temperature as you do so.

After you have run through the whole exercise programme a couple of times, you will have a pretty good idea which movements feel good and which don't seem to be doing much for you. Spend most of your time on exercises that 'hit your spots' and minimal time on the others. However, remember that you must do at least six repetitions of each exercise, except the ones that you can't do or that you have been advised to omit. People who are able to do most of the exercises in Chapters 3 and 4 may choose to omit the passive and isometric exercises in Chapter 5, which work on the same muscles and joints but require a much lower level of energy. Once you have developed enough strength and stamina to sustain a sequence of six repetitions of most of the exercises in each section, you may be assured that your programme is well rounded and might even forestall or minimize future arthritis involvement in joints not yet affected by the disease.

Be sure to keep the door to the bathroom closed when filling the bathtub and during exercise sessions if room air temperature is initially less than 75°F (24°C). This allows the air and water temperatures to stabilize, since heat tends to escape from water into the air of a cooler room. Spa and hot tub users may have less control of the surrounding air temperature because they are generally placed in a larger open area. Be sure to have a thick towel or a warm robe ready in which to wrap yourself as soon as you finish exercising, if the air is at all cool. A wet body can cause an unwelcome, unhealthy chill, and can actually prompt the return of pain or increase its severity.

Plan to exercise regularly, at least three times a week with the full programme; the other days light exercises will help alleviate stiffness. Steady progress will speed you to your goal sooner than long-drawn-out sporadic sessions. These generally accomplish little beyond fatiguing your muscles so that they tend to cramp later in the day or at night.

If you can really feel the benefit of a certain exercise, or if the exercises in a particular chapter seem to help more than the others, then that is where you should concentrate your efforts. You can do the minimum number of certain others that don't benefit you as much, but you must do a few of all of them, with the exception of wrist and finger exercises if you have no specific problem with your hands or fingers. If any exercise causes pain it should be omitted, at least temporarily, unless you have specifically been advised by your doctor or therapist to continue with it.

SUGGESTED NUMBER OF REPETITIONS

The number of repetitions of each particular exercise and the amount of time the position is held are a matter of individual conditioning and personal preference. We generally recommend that you begin with a nominal two or three repetitions and then try to work up to ten, if you can. People with arthritis who experience pain initially must exercise less vigorously or make their movements less broad.

Exercises that don't involve an affected part of your body may be very easy for you to do. You may find that you can do ten repetitions easily, almost from the beginning. You may want to go beyond ten repetitions if a particular exercise feels especially good to you. You may do as many as fifteen or even twenty after the first few days of the programme, when your body has become used to a given movement. But if you increase the number of repetitions, or the length of time (count) that you hold a particular position too quickly, you may find yourself stiff and sore several hours later. Our instructions generally tell you to hold for a count of three, and that is probably what you should do the first few times you go through the programme. Holding any position past the count of ten is not particularly recommended, because the exercise value at that point has reached its peak. The same reasoning applies to doing more than twenty repetitions of any one exercise.

A better way to increase the value of each exercise is to wear a long-sleeved cotton shirt and long trousers, or a sweatshirt and sweatpants if you really want to increase the drag. This enhances the strengthening properties of the movements, especially those requiring you to lift your hands and feet out of the water. (Remember that if you add chlorine to spa water you can expect your clothing to fade.)

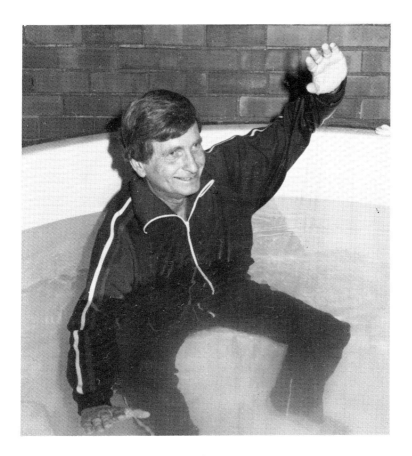

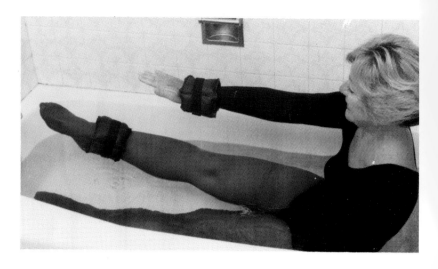

Wrist- and ankle-weights of many kinds are also available through sports or department stores. Wearing them increases the load on the muscles and joints that move your hands and feet through the water. Do not use these devices without consulting your doctor or the therapy staff.

POSITIONING YOUR BODY

Each person's body is slightly different, not only in terms of basic height and weight distribution, but also in the relative length of arms, legs and torso. Individuals also vary in their ability to bend or straighten specific areas of their body, as well as in general flexibility. Bathtubs differ remarkably in their height and width and in the slope of their backs and sides. The whole situation gets even more complicated when you compare the various spas and hot tubs available. Each manufacturer, it seems, has different standards for dimensions and configurations, and even these specifications vary from one model to another within the same brand.

Considering all these variables it is easy to understand why we cannot possibly give precise information regarding how to brace your body or how far to move your arms or legs within the limited confines of a bath and the various spas, particularly those with moulded interiors. Just follow the instructions and illustrations for each exercise as closely as you can.

Bending your knees slightly will improve your balance and

be a little easier on your back, but keeping them straight will strengthen your abdominal muscles. Of course, if your legs are long and your bath is short you will have little choice for many of the exercises unless you want to raise your legs until you are able to prop your feet against the front of the bath, while keeping your knees straight. Draping your forearms along the edges of the bath when working with your legs or feet will help to brace and steady your body. Some people will feel more secure by sliding their fingers under each buttock, backs of hands resting just to the side of the lower spine when they lean against the back wall of the bath. Try this position if bracing your hands on the bath ledge doesn't work too well for you. You may want to brace your feet, lower legs and knees against the sides of the bath while exercising your shoulders and arms, or you may find none of these special positions is even necessary in your particular case.

The important thing to remember is that if we don't specifically instruct you to put your arms or legs in a particular position, you may do whatever comes naturally and feels the most comfortable. You may even find that you are more comfortable exercising while sitting on a small, sturdy, rubber-tipped, four-legged stool. It also makes getting in and out of the bath a lot easier, and it is quite acceptable as long as you bear in mind that you won't get the same benefits of the water's buoyancy to the parts of your body that are not submerged.

You will soon develop a feeling for when you are firmly braced and when you might slip. For instance, a small person like Judy, who is five feet tall, can stretch her legs out more fully than can Bill, who measures five feet nine inches, so Judy must take a little more care when bracing herself. Nancy, who has rheumatoid arthritis, must be careful not to grip the edge of the tub because it might damage her already painful finger joints. Judy and Bill, who have no problems with their fingers or hands, can grasp the edge any way that they wish.

You may choose to angle your body sideways when performing certain exercises requiring broad lateral simultaneous arm movements if you are using a bathtub or moulded spa with high sides or where space is limited. However, if you arm span is too broad, or if flexibility in your knees or hips is limited, this position probably won't work for you. In that case just exercise one arm at a time and turn your body completely around so that you face the other way when you are ready to exercise the arm that needs more room. To avoid shifting back and forth in the tub or spa, it is better to do all of the arm exercises in two sequences – first exercise the un-encumbered arm, then shift around so the other arm is free and repeat the exercises using that arm.

Users of rounded spas or hot tubs don't generally encounter the problem of space restriction to the side, but they may have to modify the positioning of their feet since they are usually sitting on a ledge with their feet beneath their knees. Turning sideways and stretching your legs out on the ledge may be more comfortable during certain exercises.

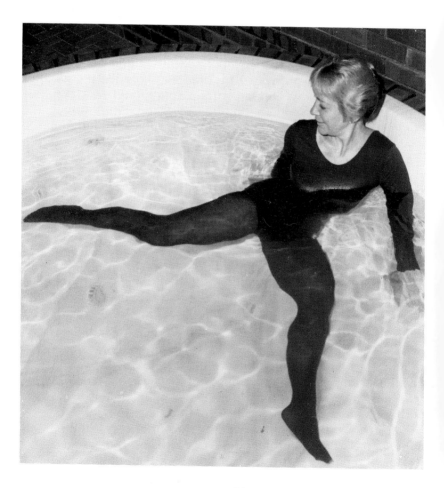

WATER DEPTH

Fill your tub or spa to armpit level, if you can, although you may want to lower the water level a few inches or so when you get to the aerobic section to avoid unnecessary splashing and to inject more difficulty into the programme. On the other hand, keeping the water level high for aerobic exercises will minimize strain on painful muscles and joints. Use your best judgement, keeping safety considerations uppermost in your mind.

Most bathtubs have a drain-overflow hole somewhere beneath the tap that prevents the water level from rising above the manufacturer's specifications. You can plug the hole with a small facecloth to allow a higher water level, but be careful not to leave the bathwater running unattended or you will end up with a flood!

BREATHING AND TIMING

Rhythmic breathing is an important part of exercise. It allows oxygen to enter your lungs and, just as important, it allows your lungs to eliminate carbon dioxide and other waste products. People who practise proper breath control experience far less cramping than those who breathe sporadically. More oxygen is supplied to your working muscles more efficiently, and your body's waste products don't have a chance to build to high levels.

Yoga practitioners have emphasized the benefits of rhythmic exercise and breath control for centuries. Today's aerobic-dancing enthusiasts take advantage of the same rhythmic principles, although in a far more vigorous manner.

Some exercises direct you to hold your position for a certain number of counts. This leads to two potential problems: (1) figuring out how fast to count; and (2) remembering to breathe. Try to make the time between each count equal to about one second. An easy way to approximate one second when no clock is handy is to say the number aloud, followed by the words 'one thousand': for example, 'one, one thousand; two, one thousand; three, one thousand,' and so on. Counting aloud actually eliminates the second problem – the need to concentrate on breathing – and frees your mind for the actual exercise. Another way to assure rhythmic breathing is to inhale while a part of your body is being extended and exhale as it is being drawn to you or returned to the starting position. Of course this method is not recommended when doing aerobic or other fast-paced movements.

Perhaps the simplest trick to maintain proper rhythmic breathing is to sing a song – a slow, romantic ballad for gentle stretching and holding exercises and something a little more lively for exercises where you have to speed up. The aerobic section can be done to tunes ranging from a John Philip Sousa march to a Michael Jackson beat.

You may have heard someone explain the benefits of breathing from the diaphragm and not understood exactly how to do it. Singing automatically ensures correct breathing if you just let go and belt it out. Don't fret about the quality of your voice or the possibility of appearing silly. After all, singing in the bath is an accepted tradition. If you don't know all the right words to a particular song, you can just make up some of your own.

EXERCISE SEQUENCE

It is not necessary to do the exercises in precisely the sequences listed, especially if you want to spend maximum time on those that feel the best or will do the most good for you. We do suggest, however, that you do a few of the exercises designed for each part of your body so that you get a total workout and that you follow the general exercise sequences as we have outlined them by chapter, unless active movement is too painful. Begin with your Pre-Session Warm-Ups in Chapter 3 before tackling the Active Limbering and Strengthening movements in Chapter 4. Continue on to the Aerobic Exercises in Chapter 6 and do whatever exercises you are able to do for whatever time you can manage without strain. Gradually increase the number of exercises and the number of repetitions as you become better conditioned. You can also do them with increased vigour or with the weights or clothing we mentioned earlier *if your doctor approves*.

Many of the exercises involve co-ordination and will be difficult to do at first. It is important that you stick with it no matter how temporarily frustrated you become. Muscle co-ordination itself is every bit as important as flexibility and strength in the maintenance or enhancement of the total quality of your life.

Always go back to Chapter 3 for a few minutes before you finish your programme. A few of the gentle stretching and strengthening movements at the end of your session, especially the favourites that felt good when you began, allow your muscles to cool down gradually so that they won't cramp later.

You can substitute the passive and isometric exercises in Chapter 5 for the active ones in Chapter 3, 4 and 6 on days when your muscles just won't function without a lot of pain. These exercises are of special benefit to people who are in extreme pain or who are paralyzed. If pain or paralysis make it difficult or even impossible to move an arm, hand, leg or foot on its own, you may find that you can lift and position that part of your body just by tucking your unimpaired arm or leg beneath it. Exercises that can be performed using passive-movement techniques are marked 'Passive' after the list of joints affected that appears below the description of the exercise.

A helper, generally another family member, can gently grasp and move a joint for you, too, if you are unable to exercise it independently.

Massage, although not exercise in the strict sense of the word, does improve blood-flow as well as feeling very good. Ideally it should be done at the very beginning or end of your programme, so that it does not hasten the cooling down of your muscles too rapidly during your workout time. Do not use massage as a substitute for the strengthening and stretching exercises in Chapters 3 and 4.

CRAMPING

Cramping, especially of toes or lower leg muscles, is a common complaint, particularly of the elderly. Cramps often come at night and seem to occur with predictable regularity. Sometimes they also hit during or after exercise. Although a thorough discussion of causes and treatments of cramps is beyond the scope of this book, it is useful to know that simple cramps in the calf or in the toes are most easily relieved by cupping the ball of your foot in your palm, fingers pointing away from your toes, and gently pressing your hand against your toes, forcing them gently upwards towards the knee. Stretching the muscles and tendons in toes and the lower leg causes the knotted muscles to relax. If you can't get your foot near enough to your hand to use this method, an alternative is to place the sole of your non-cramped foot on the tips of your toes to force them backward. Either way, increase the pressure gradually and discontinue it if you feel any pain other than the original cramp. Do not resume exercise or massage until your cramp has disappeared. It may return if you do.

Frequent cramps, although painful and annoying, are not necessarily an indication of a serious underlying condition. Still, it is best to report them if they occur frequently and let your doctor decide their relative significance. Your total health can be better evaluated if your doctor has complete information. You may be advised to eat foods rich in minerals such as calcium or potassium to relieve cramping, or you may even be given vitamins or minerals in pill form. Doctors sometimes run blood tests to determine the cause of cramping, and sometimes they merely advise cutting back on certain activities. However, many people who undertake an exercise programme report cramping much less frequently than before they began it. Just remember, if cramping persists, don't rely on the advice of family, friends, magazines or books. Let your doctor determine the cause.

WHIRLPOOL OR HYDROCIRCULATION AIRFLOW MASSAGE

Although not necessary, it is perfectly fine to do your exercises while using a whirlpool device, as long as the force of the whirlpool circulation isn't so strong that it causes any problems with your balance or is not too harsh for the painful areas of your body. Remember, in any case, that the action is massaging in nature and, although it will help circulation somewhat, it is not actual exercise and does not provide the same benefits as exercise. These devices are great to own, but don't feel that you must go out and buy one to get the maximum benefit from your water exercises.

EXERCISING IN HOT TUB AND SPA

We have illustrated most of the exercises in a bathtub because most readers do not have access to a hot tub or spa on a regular basis. The main benefit of a hot tub or spa is the extra room available to stretch arms and legs to the side. Certain types also allow the user to lie back easily so that painful joints in the upper back, shoulders and neck can be submerged while they are being working through their routine. As mentioned before, users of rounded hot tubs or spas may find certain exercises easier if they turn sideways to rest their feet on the bench seat rather than in the footwell. Just use our illustrations and your own comfort level as a guide, and do what makes the most common sense.

Users of hot tub and spa should do the exercises in sections pertaining to bathtubs, as well as those in the special hot tub and spa chapter.

SPECIAL INSTRUCTIONS FOR CERTAIN MEDICAL CONDITIONS

A few of these exercises list special precautions for people with specific medical conditions. These warnings must be strictly observed. Not to do so can cause needless pain and can even make the condition worse. For example, your neck is a very delicate area of your body. It is actually the beginning of your whole spinal column. Damage here can result in severe pain or even paralysis. We have included a few neck exercises for people who want to know how to exercise this area safely and adequately, but we strongly recommend that you use very slow and deliberate motions when doing the neck exercises and check with your doctor if you have any doubt at all about the general condition of this potentially sensitive part of your body. All exercises involving the neck are followed by a warning.

Backs are another delicate area. We have indicated which exercises may pose a problem to someone who already has back pain. These exercises should not automatically be avoided by anyone with a bad back, because it is as necessary to maintain flexibility and strength in a sore back as in a healthy one. However, it is wise to consult your doctor if you have back problems to find out which and how much of each back exercise is good for you. If you develop pain in your back while doing any of these movements, you must stop the exercise immediately. If it still hurts when you attempt it a session or two later, you should let your doctor know. Medical advice about how many repetitions to do each session and at what

21

pace the exercise should be performed must be taken seriously.

Pinned or artificial hips, knees or other joints can be damaged if special warnings are not heeded. These implants are subject to ordinary mechanical breakdown caused by undue stress, as are any other mechanical devices. Remember, too, plastic or metal joints don't need exercise as human tissue does.

Finally, we must address those with heart disease. No one should undertake a regular exercise programme without at least a general check-up that includes attention to an individual's heart and blood pressure. Only then should decisions be made about how often to exercise, how long during each session, and which specific exercises are to be emphasized or avoided. Aerobic exercises can strengthen your heart muscle, but you must ask your doctor if you should do them, for how long and, most important, how high your pulse rate can be safely elevated, especially if you have a history of heart disease. Never rely on general guidelines, even from so-called experts. Health and fitness organizations, and people within these organizations themselves, disagree on ideal pulse-rate levels during exercise. Anyone with a history of high blood pressure or heart disease would be irresponsible not to consult a doctor before undertaking any new exercise programme.

HOW TO FIND YOUR TARGET HEART RATE

Although you should take your pulse several times during your period of exercise, we particularly recommend that it be checked every five minutes while doing the aerobic exercises described in Chapter 6 to ensure that you are exercising vigorously enough to strengthen your heart, but not overdoing it to the point of potential harm. By relaxing for a minute and re-monitoring your pulse rate to find how much it has dropped, both you and your doctor will have a really good indication of your overall cardiac health. As a rule of thumb the more dramatic the drop in heart rate, the better conditioned you are.

We have prepared a table of generally recognized and accepted guidelines for target heart rates by age group on page 141, and a conversion table of ten-second heart rates to find the beats per minute on page 142, along with instructions for the use of the tables. We strongly suggest that you study these tables to get a good feel for your capabilities and limitations. *Specific instructions from your own doctor supersede the general recommendations in our tables.*

Two easy-to-find safe spots for monitoring your pulse rate are at the wrist or in the upper arm near the biceps muscle, although your pulse can also be detected as many other sites on your body. Taking your pulse at the neck is not recommended because you can interfere with the blood flow to your head.

To find the pulse in your wrist you must turn either hand palm up. Keep your wrist straight and your elbow tucked into your side. It also helps to place your wrist on your bent knee or on the edge of the tub or spa. Place the first three fingers of your other hand firmly at the base of your forearm, just beneath the crease of your wrist. Press and slide your fingers outward until they are roughly in line with your thumb. You will feel the pulsation beneath one or two of your fingers as you move away from the centre of your forearm. Never use your thumb to feel for a pulse. If you can't find your pulse using one wrist, try changing hands and searching for it in the other.

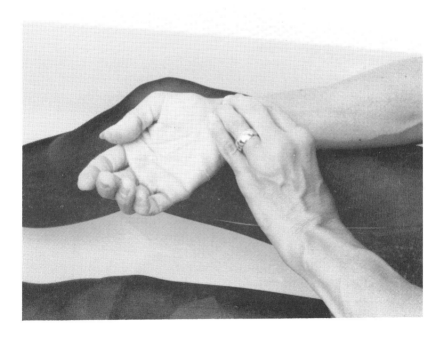

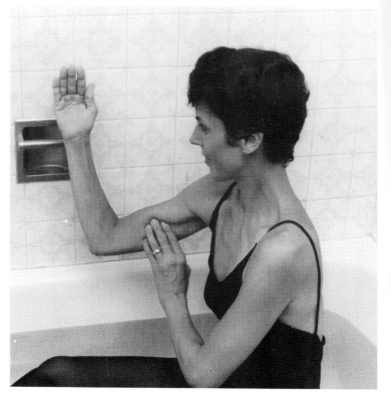

You have an even stronger pulse in your upper arm. To find it raise and extend either upper arm until your elbow is about level with your nipples. Rest it on your raised knees or at the side of the bath, palm up. Press the fingers of your other hand firmly against your upper arm, just before the spot where your biceps muscle begins to bulge – a little higher than half-way between your elbow and your armpit. You will be pressing on your humerus bone. Your pulse can be felt in the crease just next to it on the lower inside of your arm. You may have to walk your fingers around the general area the first few times to hit just the right spot.

If you are unsuccessful in finding either of these pulse spots, ask your doctor or one of the staff to help. It is a very good idea to practise finding your pulse during a quiet time out of water. Don't become frustrated if you don't succeed the first few times, even after some assistance. Just keep plugging away and you'll be successful eventually.

3

Pre-Session Warm-Up

Gentle stretching exercises loosen stiff muscles and joints and allow for freer movement without risk to sore areas. Conversely, starting an exercise session with vigorous strengthening or aerobic movements can actually cause physical damage. Exercises in this section can be done easily in a deep spa, but conventional bathtub exercisers will find it difficult to submerge active body parts deep enough to get maximum benefit. However, the exercises can be done while standing or, perhaps, sitting on a sturdy stool under a running shower directed at the shoulders so that the warm moist heat and gentle massaging action of the water will work directly on neck, shoulder and back muscles, while the plugged bath fills for the main exercise sequences.

The exercises in this section have been illustrated in the standing position, but it is obvious that the same movements can be performed by anyone sitting on a stool or in the bath.

1. Shoulder Circles

Circle your left shoulder to the front, then up, back, and then around to the front again. Make the circle as full as you can without pain. Repeat. Reverse direction. Repeat with your right shoulder. Now circle them both simultaneously, first forwards and then backwards.

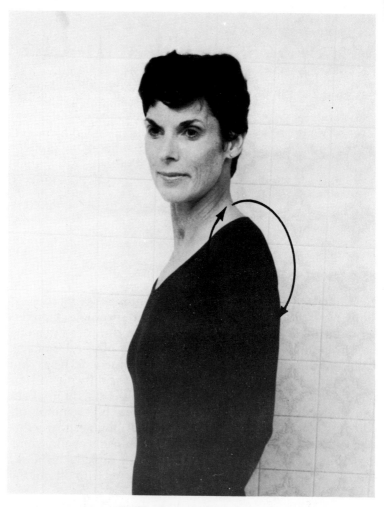

☐ Neck/Shoulders/Upper Back

2. Split the Rail

Imagine you are holding an axe in your hands. Raise your straight arms overhead and then bend forward as you swing your clasped hands downwards vigorously, as if chopping a block of wood. If you are sitting in the bath, you may spread your knees and bring your hands all the way down to the bottom of the bath, if you don't mind the splash. Otherwise, stop just above the waterline. Repeat.

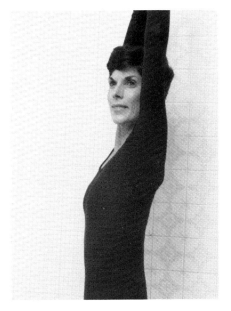

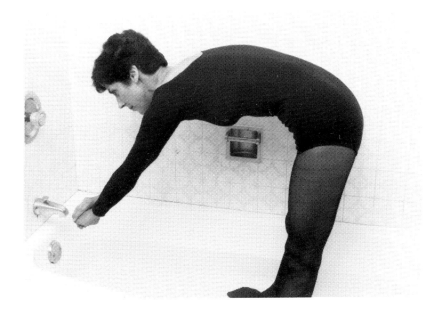

☐ Shoulders/Lower Back/Hips/Passive

27

3. Arm Swing

Stretch both arms out to the side and move them behind your body as far as you can while still keeping them straight. Your fingers are together. Try to keep your arms as high as possible at all times. Arc your arms past the front of your body, letting them cross until they can go no farther without bending at the elbow. Then swing your arms back to the original position. Repeat.

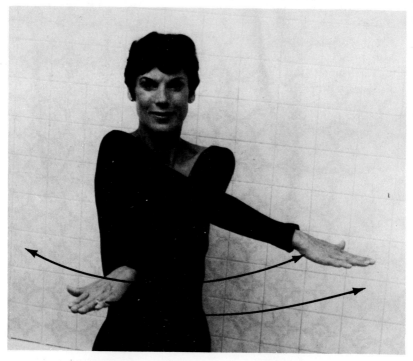

☐ Shoulders

CAUTION: *People with shoulder replacements or pins must not move their wrists on the affected side past the midpoint of their bodies.*

4. Torso Stretch

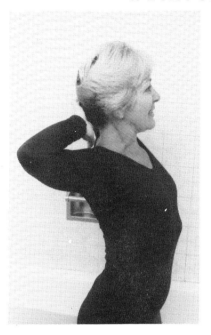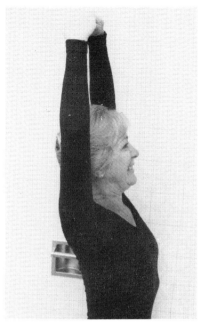

Clasp your hands behind your neck, or just put one hand on top of the other, if you find that position more comfortable. Straighten your elbows to raise your hands as high overhead as you can, palms to the ceiling. Stretch your torso upwards so that your hands reach even higher. Hold for a count of three, and then return your hands to behind your neck. Repeat.

☐ Shoulders/Torso/Elbows/Wrists/Passive

5. Cross Your Heart Twice

Put the fingers of your left hand on the tip of your right shoulder. Cross your right forearm over your left forearm and let the fingers of your right hand touch your left shoulder. Be very sure to keep your shoulders relaxed and your elbows as close to your body as is comfortable. Now uncross your arms and put your hands behind your back, trying to cross your left wrist over your right wrist near the middle of your back. Your palms point away from your body and your fingertips point at your shoulderblades. (Don't be discouraged if you find this difficult. Just do your best and get your hands as far up your back as you can without pain.) Uncross your wrists and recross your heart, this time with the left forearm passing over the right. Then move your hands to the rear and cross your right wrist over your left. Repeat, alternating top arm and wrist each time.

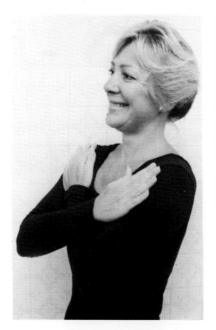 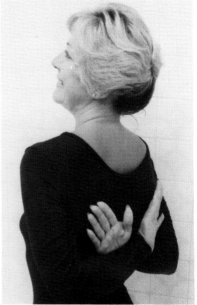

☐ Shoulders/Elbows

CAUTION: *People with surgical shoulder replacements must not cross their hands to the rear.*

6. Double Twist

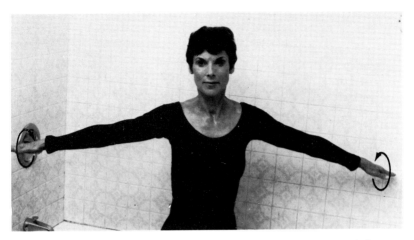

Angle your body so that you can stretch both arms straight out to the side, palms down, fingers spread. If your bath is too narrow to allow you to use both arms simultaneously, just work with one at a time. Inhale and clench your fists as you rotate your palms until they face the ceiling. Exhale as you reverse the rotation and straighten your fingers. Repeat.

☐ Shoulders/Upper Back/Upper Arms/Fingers

7. Palms to the Ceiling

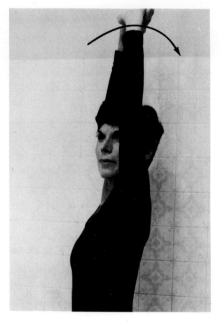

Lift your arms directly over-head, or as high as you can get them comfortably. Your elbows must be straight. Both palms face the ceiling, one beneath the other. Stretch your torso upwards as if trying to touch the ceiling with your palms. Now bring your straight arms backwards as far as you can. Ideally your upper arms will be behind your ears. Return your arms to the upright position, hold for a count of three, then relax your torso, keeping your hands elevated. Repeat.

☐ Shoulders/Torso/Lower Back/Passive

CAUTION: *Discontinue this exercise if you experience any discomfort in your back.*

8. Upsy-Daisy

Interlace your fingers behind your back, palms facing one another. Bend forward slightly as you lift both arms behind you. Keep your elbows as straight as you can. Hold for a count of three, and return your hands to the starting position. Repeat.

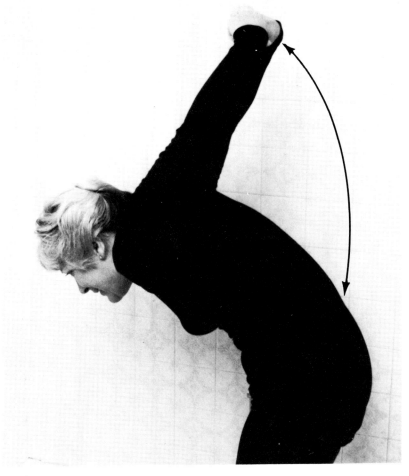

☐ Shoulders/Lower Back/Abdomen

CAUTION: *People with surgical shoulder replacements must omit this exercise.*

9. Behind the Back

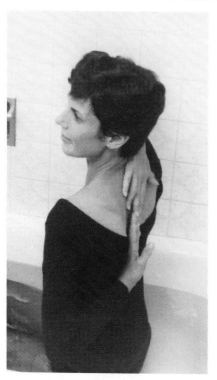

Sit straight and bring your right hand over your right shoulder and down your spine as far as you can. At the same time bend your left elbow and put your left hand behind your back, moving it up your spine as high as possible. Try to get the fingers of each hand to touch. Relax. Repeat. Reverse the position of your hands so that the left one passes its shoulder to stretch downwards and the right one goes behind your back to meet the left. Repeat. Don't be upset if the fingers of one hand don't touch those of the other behind you. Most people's won't.

☐ Shoulders/Elbows/Torso

CAUTION: *People with surgical shoulder replacements must omit this exercise.*

10. Neck Swivel

Keep your head level throughout this exercise. Turn your head to the left as far as is comfortable, letting your eyes follow along with this smooth and controlled movement. Pause. Now swing your head as far to the right as you can. Pause. Repeat.

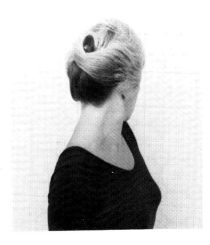 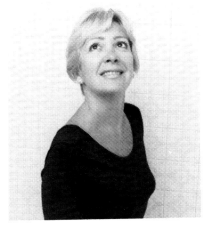

☐ Neck

CAUTION: *Repeated head movement may cause slight dizziness. Be sure to steady yourself by bracing a hand against a wall or other stationary object, particularly if you are standing. The neck is an extremely sensitive body area and must be treated delicately. If any indication of medical abnormality exists, we strongly recommend that you check with your doctor before performing this exercise.*

11. Nod a 'V'

Turn your head to the left as far as you can comfortably and raise your chin. As you move your head to the centre of your body drop your chin until it nears or contacts your chest. Raise your chin again as your head moves to the extreme right. This motion traces the letter V. Your eyes must follow the movement of your head. Repeat. Reverse the motion, beginning at the right and moving left. Repeat.

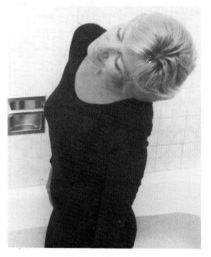 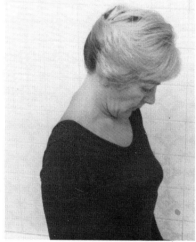

☐ Neck

CAUTION: *Repeated head movement may cause slight dizziness. Be sure to steady yourself by bracing a hand against a wall or other stationary object, particularly if you are standing. The neck is an extremely sensitive body area and must be treated delicately. If any indication of medical abnormality exists, we strongly recommend that you check with your doctor before performing this exercise.*

12. Drop and Roll

Drop your right ear as if trying to touch it to your shoulder, but do not raise your shoulder at all. Your left ear will be pointed directly towards the ceiling. Now drop your chin to your chest and roll your head as far to the left as you can, being sure to end the movement with your right ear to the ceiling. Pause. Reverse the motion, beginning on the left and moving to the right. Pause. Repeat the sequence.

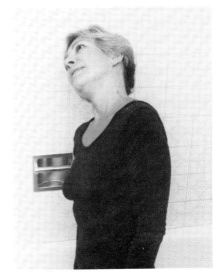

☐ Neck

CAUTION: *Repeated head movement may cause slight dizziness. Be sure to steady yourself by bracing a hand against a wall or other stationary object, particularly if you are standing. The neck is an extremely sensitive body area and must be treated delicately. If any indication of medical abnormality exists, we strongly recommend that you check with your doctor before performing this exercise.*

4

Active Limbering and Strengthening

These exercises may be done when your muscles and joints feel good enough for active movement. If these movements hurt too much or if you simply do not have the ability to handle the range of motion or degree of strength necessary, just bypass this chapter and go on to the next, which outlines passive limbering and strengthening exercises, until you develop enough flexibility and strength to attempt these again.

When working through the exercises in this chapter we suggest that you sit down and lean against the back of the bathtub or spa for support, unless we specifically call for a different position. However, if you feel that you need a more extensive workout for your abdominal muscles you may sit up straight with your back away from the wall while you perform your routine. Bending your knees slightly will improve your balance, but keeping them straight increases abdominal strength. People with problems involving the lower back may experience pain in this position, however, and should exercise cautiously with straight legs. Draping your forearms along the edges of the tub when possible will also help you to brace and steady yourself.

Spa and hot tub users may assume a sitting position with their feet beneath them, stretching their straight, unsupported legs out in front of their bodies during certain exercises. This position allows more room for sideways motion, but it puts more tension on the abdominal muscles. An alternative position is to turn sideways and place your legs on the seat beside you. Your range of movement is somewhat restricted on the side next to the spa wall, but you can do the movements using the unencumbered arm or leg first, then turn 180° and exercise the other side of your body.

13. Hand Synchronization

Keep your elbows at your waist as you face your submerged palms towards one another, fingers together, forearms parallel to your thighs. Bend your wrists by pointing the fingers of both hands to the left and then to the right. Don't move your elbows or forearms. Repeat.

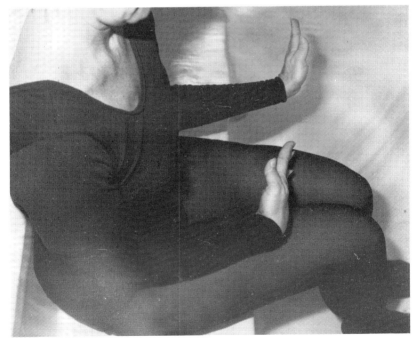

☐ Wrists/Co-ordination/Passive

14. Feet Synchronization

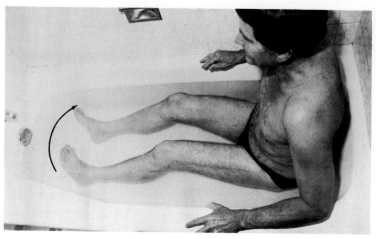

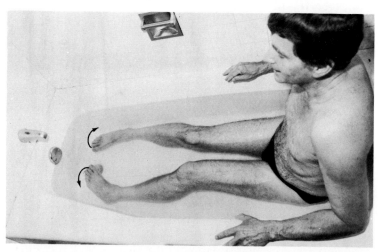

Face forward with your legs extended. Turn both feet as far as you can to the right so that the outside edge of your right foot and the inside edge of your left foot rest on or near the bottom of the bath. Now rotate both feet in the other direction so the outside edge of your left foot and the inside edge of your right foot rest on or near the bottom. Repeat. Finally, point each foot towards the other and then away as far as possible in opposite directions. Repeat.

☐ Hips/Ankles/Co-ordination

15. Double-Digit Synchronization

Face forward, brace yourself firmly, and extend your legs. Point your hands and feet simultaneously, first to the right and then to the left. Repeat. Now point the fingers and toes of each hand and foot towards the other and then away. Repeat.

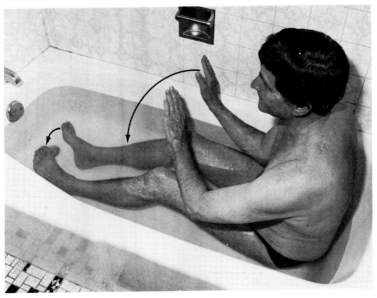

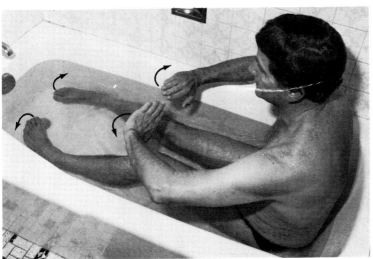

☐ Wrists/Ankles/Hips/Co-ordination

16. Finger Swinger

Sit with your knees spread wide. Submerge your hands between your knees, elbows straight and palms facing down. Bend your wrists letting your straight fingers drop until the backs of your hands face the floor. Your fingers parallel the bottom. Keep your wrists at the same depth as you slowly raise your straight fingers until they point upwards as high as possible. Hold for a count of three. You'll feel a great deal of tension through your forearms and wrists. Repeat. Now alternate the direction of your hands by bending your right wrist downwards while the fingers of your left hand point up. Reverse the action. Hold for a count of three each time. Repeat.

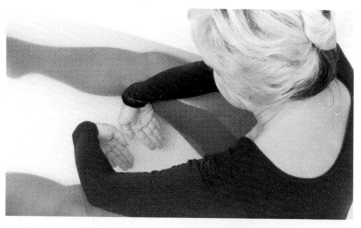

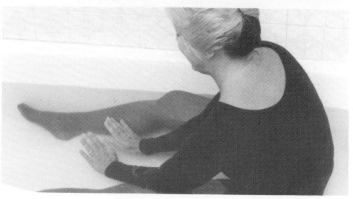

☐ Wrists/Fingers/Passive

17. Foot Flaps

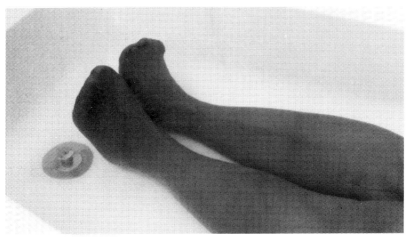

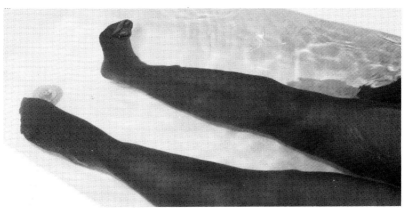

Sit comfortably. You may spread your knees. Point your toes to the ceiling or even towards your face if you are able, and hold for a count of three. You'll feel a pulling sensation in your calves. Lower your toes slowly until they point as far forward as possible. Hold for another count of three. Repeat. Now alternate the direction of your feet by pointing the left forward and the right towards your body. Hold for a count of three, then reverse the positions so that your right foot points forward and the left towards your body. Hold for a count of three. Repeat.

☐ Lower Legs/Ankles/Co-ordination

18. Swing and Flap

This exercise combines all the movements of the previous two. Place your hands between your knees. Begin by simultaneously pointing your hands and feet up and then down, just as before. Hold for a count of three each time. Repeat. Now point your right hand and foot up while your left hand and foot are in the down position. Reverse so that the left hand and foot are up and the right hand and foot down. Repeat, holding for a count of three.

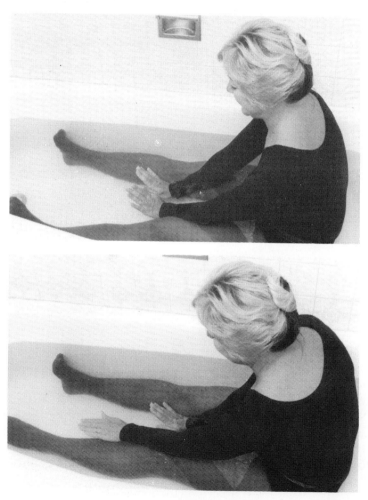

☐ Wrists/Fingers/Lower Legs/Ankles/Co-ordination

19. Horizontal Circles

Your elbows stay near your sides, forearms extended forward and parallel to the bottom of the bath. You may cup your hands and flex your wrists slightly, but keep your fingers together. Simultaneously circle both wrists to the left horizontally. Repeat. Reverse so they circle right. Repeat. Now circle both hands towards one another, repeat, and then reverse the motion so they circle away from one another. Repeat. It's OK to splash your chest with water.

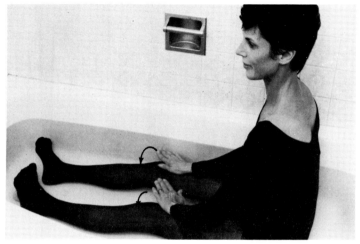

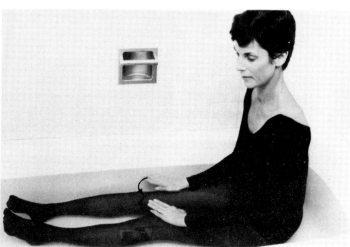

☐ Elbows/Wrists/Co-ordination

20. Rotating Palms

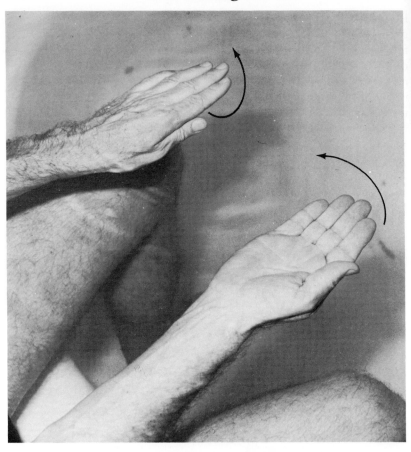

Tuck your elbows into your waist at each side. Be sure your hands and elbows are under the water. Keep your fingers straight and together as you turn the palm of your right hand upwards while your left palm faces the floor. Slowly turn your wrists so the right palm faces the floor. Slowly turn your wrists so the right palm is downwards and the left is up. Rotate again to the original position. Repeat.

☐ Elbows/Passive

21. Ankle Circles

Imagine that you have a waterproof marking-pen between the great and second toes of each foot. Simultaneously circle both feet to the right as if to draw two big round circles on the wall of the bath in front of you. Repeat. Reverse the motion and circle to the left. Repeat. Now, circle your feet inwards by turning your ankles towards each other, again drawing two imaginary circles. Repeat. Next, reverse the motion by turning your ankles outwards. Repeat.

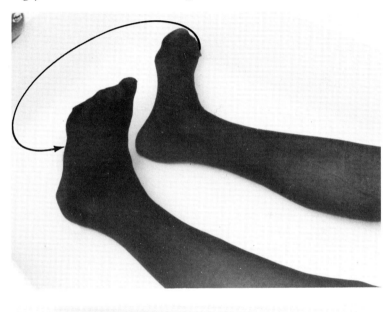

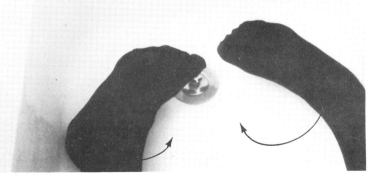

☐ Lower Legs/Ankles/Co-ordination

22. Wrist and Ankle Circles

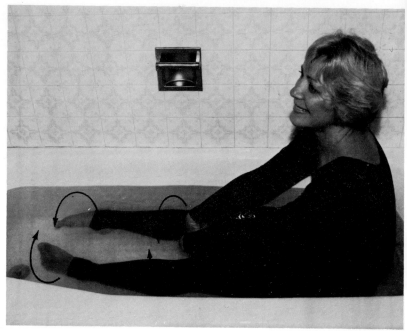

Simultaneously circle both wrists and both ankles inwards towards one another. Repeat. Now circle your wrists and ankles outwards, away from one another. Repeat.

☐ Wrists/Elbows/Lower Legs/Ankles/Co-ordination

23. Toe Holds

Place feet flat on the floor of the bath. Raise and hold your great toes as high in the air as you can. The other toes will spread out automatically. Now curl and hold your great toes beneath the balls of your feet, but do not raise your feet any higher than is absolutely necessary. The rest of your toes will bend, too. Repeat.

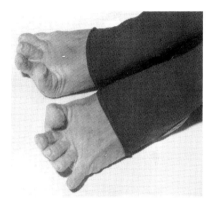 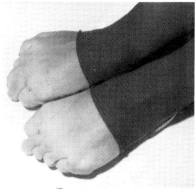

☐ Feet/Toes/Passive

24. Toe Walk

Position your body so that your feet rest flat against the floor of the bath. Now imagine that you are squeezing the floor with your toes. Hold and release. Repeat. Your foot may move forward a bit with each repetition.

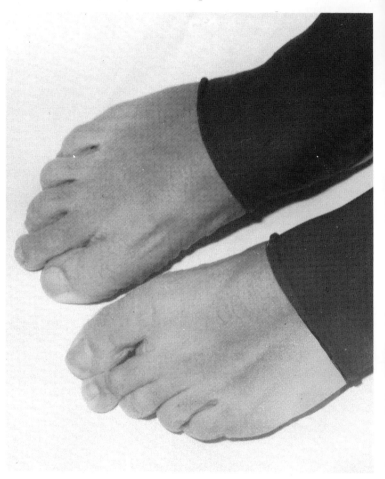

☐ Feet/Toes

25. Thumb Cross

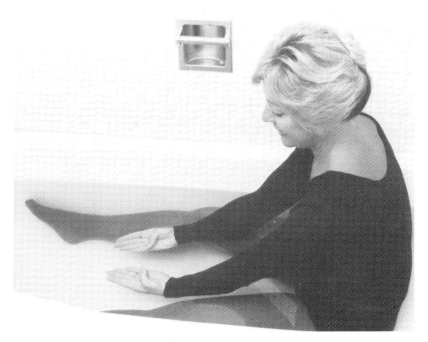

Spread your knees comfortably and submerge your out-stretched arms between your knees until your fingers are just above the bottom, palms up, fingers straight. Cross each thumb over its palm until it reaches the base of the little finger. Try not to cup your hands. Return thumbs to starting position. Cross thumbs over the palm again and put each one at the base of its ring finger. Return to original position, then cross thumbs to the middle fingers. Return thumbs again to starting position, then cross them to the base of the index fingers. Repeat sequence.

☐ Hands/Fingers/Passive

26. Thumbing the Joints

Submerge your hands between your knees. Make a palm-up fist with your right hand, making sure your thumb is outside your curled fingers. Try to place your thumb on the tip of the middle joint of the little finger. Your left hand is open, fingers straight and spread as wide as possible. Reverse your hand positions. Repeat.

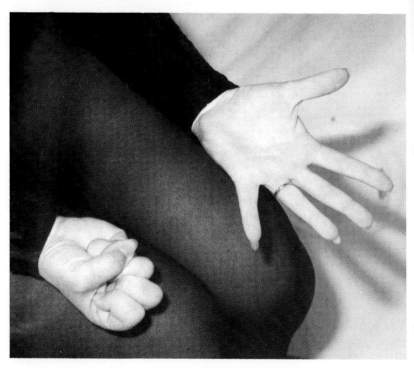

☐ Hands/Fingers/Passive

27. The Squeeze Play

Partially submerge a balled-up facecloth with your right hand, grasping it as tightly as you can comfortably. The fingers of your left hand are straight and spread wide. Release the cloth from your right hand and quickly grasp it tightly with your left hand before it drops to the bottom. The fingers of your right hand are now spread. Repeat. Keep both hands submerged at all times as you try to develop a speedy rhythm.

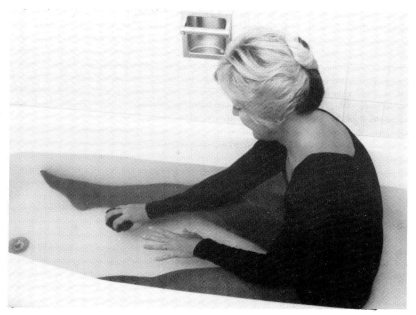

☐ Hands/Fingers/Co-ordination

28. Toe Pickup

Put your left foot over the corner of a flattened facecloth, or hold it with your toes if it is more comfortable. Try to keep it close to the bottom of the bath. Now, by curling the toes of your right foot, pick it up. When you have it grasped securely, release the pressure of your left foot and raise the cloth up to the water-line, or out of the water if you are able. You may bend your knee, but a straight leg will provide more strengthening of abdominal muscles. Return the cloth to the bottom of the bath and repeat, this time grasping the cloth with the toes of your left foot while your right foot holds it down. Repeat, alternating feet.

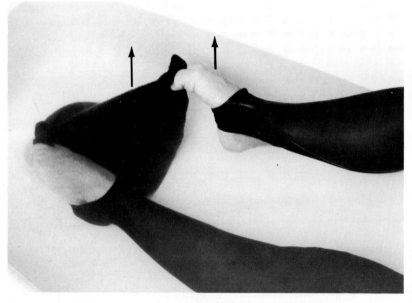

☐ Abdomen/Lower Legs/Toes

CAUTION: *You may wish to omit this exercise if you suffer from frequent foot cramping.*

29. Toe Touch

Sit upright and place your hands on your knees. Bend forward and touch the tips of your toes. The motion is slow and deliberate. Do not bounce forward. Return to the upright position with your hands on your knees. Repeat. You may eventually be able to go past your toes and touch the bottom of the bath's front wall.

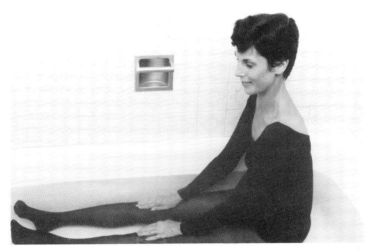

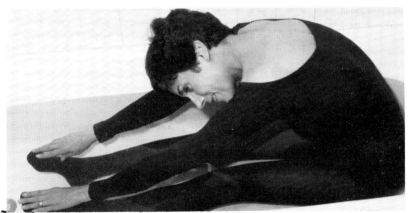

☐   Torso/Waist/Lower Back/Abdomen/Upper Legs/ Passive

CAUTION: *People with low-back pain must keep their knees slightly bent during this exercise.*

30. Touch with a Twist

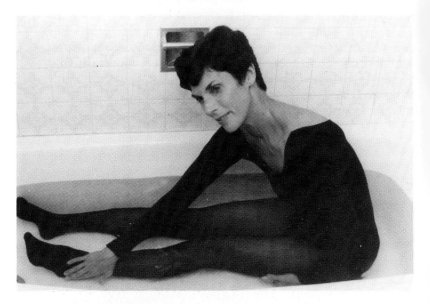

Sit upright and place your right hand on your left knee. Bend forward and touch the outside of your left ankle. The motion is slow and deliberate. Return to the upright position. Repeat exercise, this time using your left hand to touch your right knee and then right ankle. Repeat, alternating left and right ankles.

☐ Torso/Waist/Lower Back/Abdomen/Upper Legs/ Passive

CAUTION: *People with low-back pain must keep their knees slightly bent during this exercise.*

31. Touch Times Three

Spread and extend your feet directly in front of you, knees as straight as possible. Point your toes to the ceiling. Interlock your fingers and extend your straight arms to the front, palms facing away. You may place the palm of one hand on the back of the other rather than interlocking fingers, if this position is more comfortable. Bend forward and try to touch the toes of your right foot. If you can't reach your toes, just touch the place on your leg, ankle or foot that you can reach. Return to the upright position. Bend and touch the bath floor between your feet at the front of the bath. Sit up again, and then bend and touch the toes of your left foot. Return to the upright position, then bend and touch between your feet, and then back again to the toes of your right foot. Repeat the sequence. You'll feel a pulling sensation in the backs of your thighs and calves if your legs are completely straight.

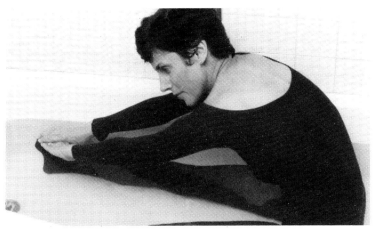

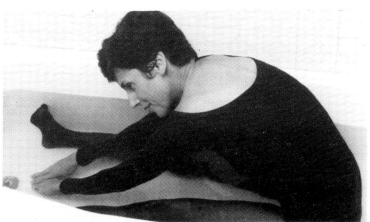

☐　　Shoulders/Torso/Waist/Abdomen/Lower Back/ Upper Legs/Lower Legs

CAUTION: *Discontinue this exercise if you experience any discomfort in your back.*

32. Easy Waist-Twisters

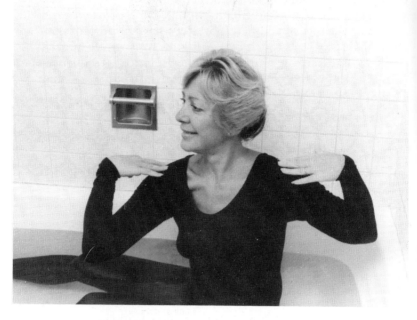

With your legs extended, lift your forearms and put your fingertips on the outside tips of your shoulders. If the space next to your bath is too narrow to allow you to touch your fingertips to the outside of your shoulders, you may touch the front of your shoulders instead. Keep your shoulders as far back as you can. Gently twist your torso to the left as far as you can. Reverse direction and twist as far to the right as possible. Repeat. Do not use bouncing or jerky motions.

☐ Waist/Torso/Lower Back

CAUTION: *People with low-back pain must twist only as far as they can without pain. They may choose to omit this exercise entirely.*

33. Twist and Touch

Sit up and twist to the left so that your right hand approaches or touches the wall behind your left shoulder. Face forward again, and then twist to the right, touching your left hand to the wall. Repeat, alternating sides. Do not use bouncing or jerky motions.

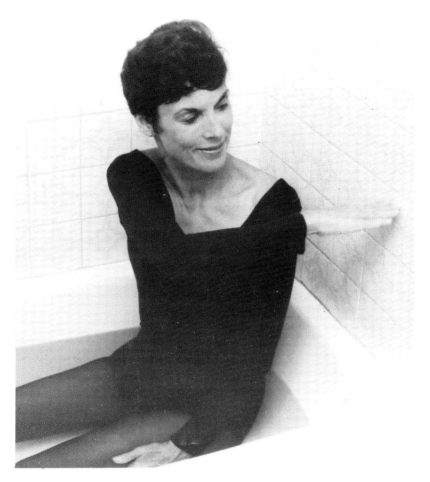

☐ Shoulders/Torso/Waist/Lower Back

CAUTION: *People with low-back pain must twist only as far as they can without pain. They may choose to omit this exercise entirely.*

34. Jelly Roll

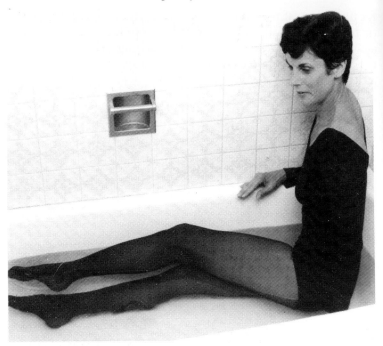

Keeping your legs as close together as you can, tighten your abdominal muscles as you roll side to side on your hips. You may raise your leg as well as your hip as you roll. You may also want to grasp the sides of the bath for balance. Don't forget to breathe. Repeat.

☐ Torso/Waist/Lower Back

CAUTION: *People with low-back pain must twist only as far as they can without pain. They may choose to omit this exercise entirely.*
Do not roll on to an artificial or pinned hip.

35. Rocking Horse

Bend your knees to your chest and grasp the underside of each thigh. Tighten your abdominal muscles as you keep your knees close to your chest and rock backwards on to your buttocks. Your feet will leave the ground. Repeat, remembering to breathe regularly. Be very careful not to rock backwards so far that you slip.

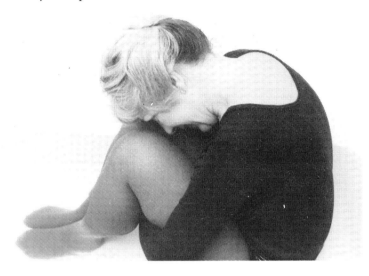

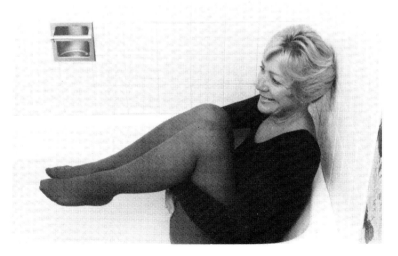

☐ Abdomen

36. Alternate Knees to Chest

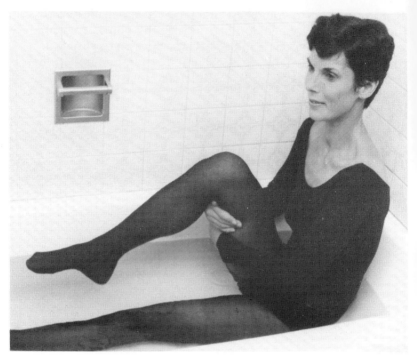

Sit up comfortably and bend your right knee towards your chest. Your left leg remains relaxed. Grasp the underside of your thigh. Your lower leg is free and your foot may move off the bottom of the bath. Pull your knee to your chest, hold for a count of three, and relax. Repeat, alternating right and left legs.

☐ Abdomen/Hips/Knees

CAUTION: *People with an artificial knee or hip, or with a pin at a hip joint, must* not *pull the affected leg forward with their hands.*

37. Knees towards Chest

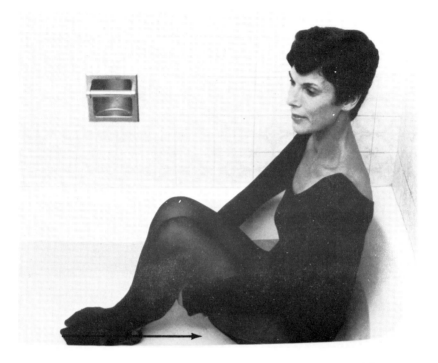

Sit up and extend your legs to the front, keeping your ankles and knees together. Grasp your thighs just behind the knees to pull your legs towards your body. Tighten your abdominal muscles as you slowly slide your feet towards your body until your knees are close to your chest. Your feet will not leave the ground. Do not lean forward, and keep your back straight. Hold this position for a count of three, then slide your feet back to the extended position. Repeat.

☐ Abdomen/Hips/Knees/Passive

CAUTION: *People with an artificial knee or hip, or a pin at a hip joint, must not pull the affected leg forward with their hands.*

38. Knee to Forehead

Lean forward and grasp your right ankle with both hands. Your left leg remains comfortably on the bottom of the bath. Straighten your right knee as you lift it to the top of the water, or even higher if you can. Bend your knee as you gently pull it up to your face. At the same time bend your neck and upper spine until your forehead touches your knee. Don't be discouraged if your forehead and knee refuse to meet. Many people are unable to close the gap. Repeat, and then do the same thing with your left leg. Be sure to return your foot to the bottom of the bath each time.

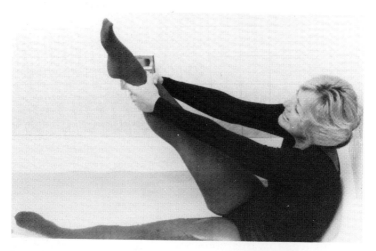

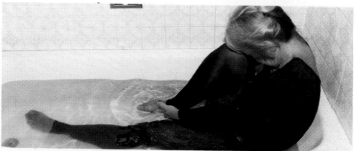

☐ Neck/Upper Back/Abdomen/Hips/Knees

CAUTION: *People with an artificial knee or hip, or a pin at a hip joint, must not pull the affected leg forward with their hands.*

39. Knee Lifts

Brace your back against the bath and your forearms against the edges as you rotate your right hip upwards and keep it there. Bend your right knee and lift it towards your chin, then straighten your leg as it returns to the bottom of the bath. Repeat, this time lifting your knee towards your left ear. Continue. Repeat the exercise with your left hip and knee.

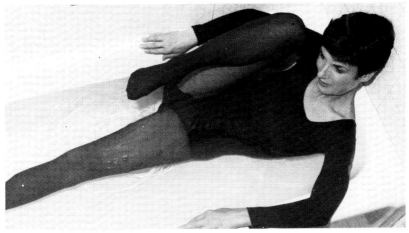

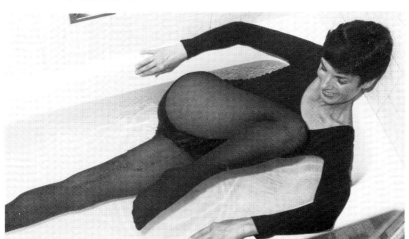

☐ Torso/Waist/Abdomen/Hips/Knees

CAUTION: *Discontinue this exercise if you experience any discomfort in your back.*

40. The Hip-Socket Roll

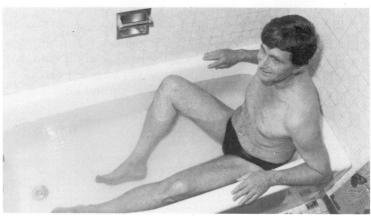

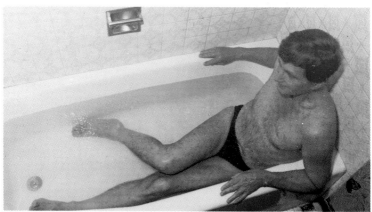

Bend your right knee so that your right foot rests flat on the bottom of the bath. Now point your knee out as you turn your foot so that its outside edge rests on or near the bottom of the bath. Roll your knee and foot in the other direction so that the inside edge of your foot rests on or near the floor. Your knee will point inwards. You may shift your foot from one side of the bath to the other so that you have more room to manoeuvre your knee back and forth. Repeat. Change to the left leg and repeat the exercise.

☐ Ankles/Hips

CAUTION: *People with an artificial hip, or a pin at their hip joint, must not do this exercise on that side.*

41. Elbow Touch

Sit forward so that you don't bump your elbows when you swing them. Clasp your hands behind your neck and touch your elbows in front of your body. Now unclasp your hands and swing your elbows to the rear, trying to touch them behind your back. You won't be able to touch your elbows at the rear, but try it anyway. Repeat.

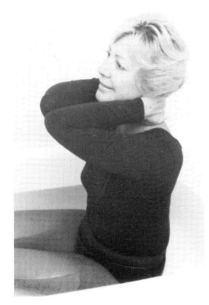 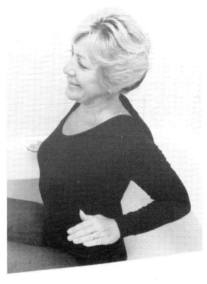

☐ Shoulders/Upper Back

CAUTION: *People with shoulder replacements or pins must discontinue this exercise if they experience pain.*

42. Rolling Pin

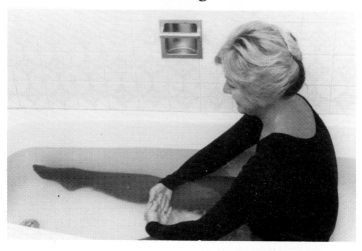

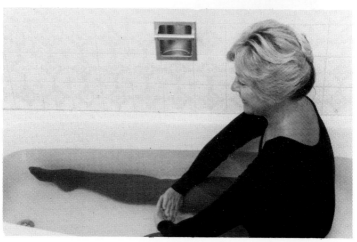

Keeping your hands underwater at all times, extend your arms forward, elbows straight, wrists bent, and palms towards your body. Interlace your fingers, or place one hand on top of the other. Bring your hands to your abdomen, rotate them so that your palms face away from you, and then straighten your elbows again as you push the water away. Rotate your wrists so that your palms face towards you again, and repeat.

☐ Shoulders/Elbows/Upper Back

43. Front Kick

Sit straight with your legs extended. Slowly lift your right foot to the surface of the water, straightening your knee as much as you can. Try to lift your heel actually out of the water. Hold for a count of three, then lower it gently back down to the bottom. Repeat. Repeat the exercise, this time lifting your left foot. This exercise should be done as slowly as possible for maximum benefit.

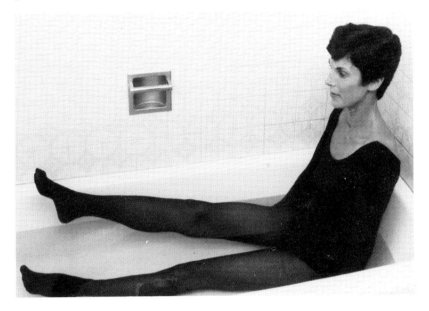

☐ Abdomen/Hips/Passive

44. Leg Lifts and Swings

Lean against the back of the bath and lift your extended right foot to the top of the water, or out of the water if you can. Try to straighten your knee. Your left foot remains comfortably on the bottom of the bath. You may grasp the sides of the bath for balance, but don't let your arm muscles substitute for your abdominal muscles when it comes to lifting your leg. Swing your raised right foot to the right as far as you can, and then to the left as far as possible. Return to the centre and lower it to the bottom of the bath. Be sure your buttocks remain firmly on the floor of the bath at all times. Repeat. Switch to the left leg, and repeat the exercise. For additional benefit, sit up straight when you perform these movements. This exercise should be done as slowly as possible for maximum benefit.

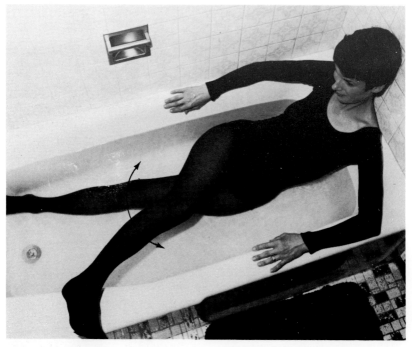

☐ Abdomen/Hips/Upper Legs

CAUTION: *Discontinue this exercise if you experience any discomfort in your back.*

People with hip replacements or pins must not move the foot of the affected leg past the mid point of their bodies.

45. Kick Lift

Grasp the sides of the bath for balance only. Bend your right knee towards your right shoulder as you lift your foot to the top of the water, or higher if you can. Now straighten your leg and hold for a count of three. Your abdominal muscles will tighten considerably. Bend your knee again and return your leg to the bottom of the bath. Repeat. Do the exercise with your left leg. Repeat. This exercise should be done as slowly as possible for maximum benefit.

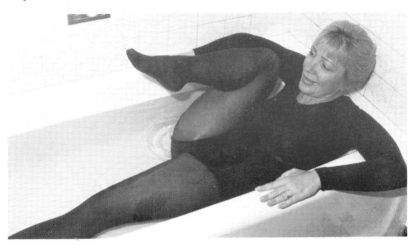

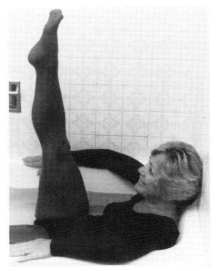

☐　Abdomen/Hips/ Upper Legs/Knees

CAUTION: People with low-back pain must keep their knees slightly bent during this exercise. Discontinue the exercise entirely if you experience pain.

46. Up and Out

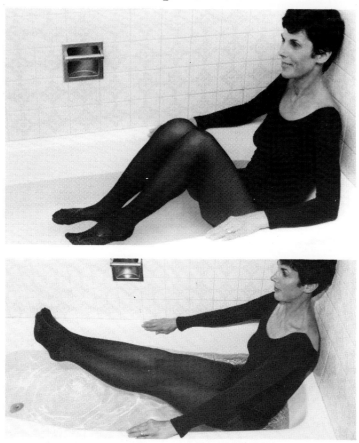

Grasp the sides of the bath for balance, if you wish, as you draw your knees towards your chest as far as you can comfortably. Now lift your feet several inches off the bottom of the bath and extend them straight out in front of you. Raise them as high as you can without discomfort. People who are in top shape will break the waterline with their heels. Hold for a count of three. Do not lean forward. Return to the bent-knee position, and then drop your feet to the bottom of the bath. Repeat. For added benefit you may stretch your arms straight out to the front as you extend your legs, but be very careful not to slip.

☐ Abdomen/Hips/Knees

47. Easy 8s

Grasp the sides of the bath for balance, if you wish, and imagine a blackboard just in front of your right foot. A waterproof marker extends out from between your toes. You may bend your knee if necessary. Raise your right foot several inches off the bottom of the bath and trace and retrace the number 8, raising your heel out of the water if you can at the top of the figure, and brushing it on the bottom of the bath at the bottom of the figure 8. Make the 8 full enough so that your foot touches each side of the tub. Repeat. Reverse direction and repeat. Switch to your left foot and repeat the sequence.

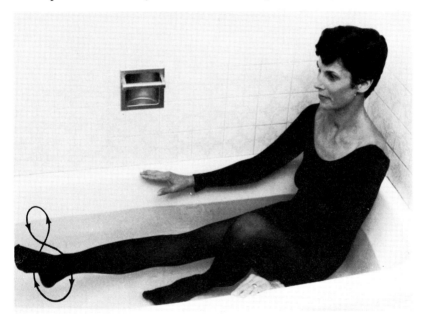

☐ Abdomen/Hips/Upper Legs

CAUTION: *People with hip replacements or pins must not move the foot of the affected leg past the midpoint of their bodies.*

48. Lazy 8s

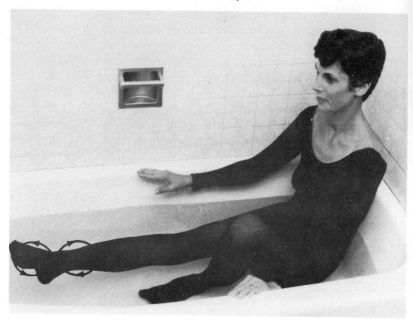

Grasp the sides of the bath for balance, if you wish, as you imagine the marker still between the toes of your right foot. Now imagine further that the *8* has toppled over on to its side. Draw this lazy *8*. Repeat. Reverse direction and repeat. Change legs and repeat the figure in both directions.

☐ Abdomen/Hips/Upper Legs

CAUTION: *People with hip replacements or pins must not move the foot of the affected leg past the midpoint of their bodies.*

49. 8s the Hard Way

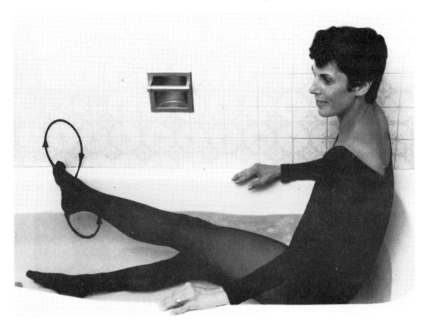

Turn on to your right hip so that the outside of your left thigh is parallel to the top of the water. You may grasp the sides of the bath for balance, if you wish. The imaginary marker is between the toes of your left foot as you again trace the number *8* in front of you. Repeat, then reverse the figure. Change legs and repeat the *8* in both directions.

☐ Abdomen/Hips/Upper Legs

CAUTION: *People with hip replacements or pins must not move the foot of the affected leg past the midpoint of their bodies.*

50. Lazy 8s the Hard Way

Turn on to your right hip again so that the outside of your left thigh is parallel to the top of the water. Continue to grasp the sides of the bath, if you wish. Again, imagine that your *8* has toppled on to its side as it did in exercise 48. Trace the *8* the usual number of repetitions, then reverse the figure and repeat. Turn on to your left hip and trace the figure with your right foot, first in one direction and then in reverse.

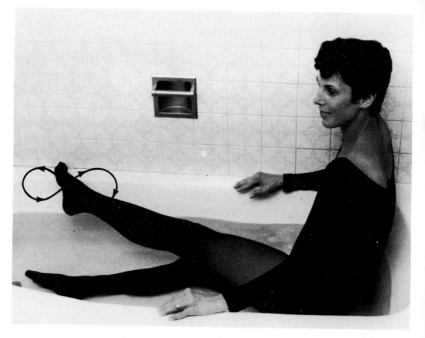

☐ Abdomen/Hips/Upper Legs

CAUTION: *People with hip replacements or pins must not move the foot of the affected leg past the midpoint of their bodies.*

51. Ankle Lifts

Grasp the sides of the bath for balance as you rotate your body so that your right hip is towards the ceiling. Lift your slightly bent right leg about six inches from the bottom of the tub, or higher if possible. Now bring your left ankle up so that it approaches or touches the right. Hold for a count of three, if you can, and then relax. Repeat. Turn on to your right hip and repeat the exercise.

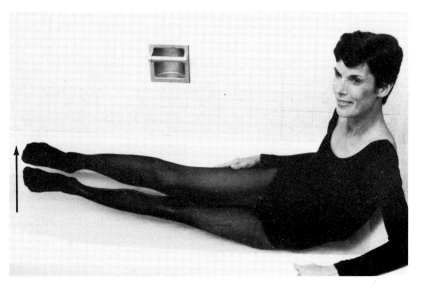

☐ Waist/Abdomen/Hips/Upper Legs

CAUTION: *People with hip replacements or pins must not move the foot of the affected leg past the midpoint of their bodies.*

People with low-back pain must keep their knees slightly bent during this exercise, or omit it entirely for a while.

5

Passive Limbering and Strengthening

The exercises in this chapter limber and strengthen muscles and joints that are paralysed or that are too sore or weak to move actively under their own power. Maintaining strength and motion where possible is important, not only to help limit or prevent pain but also to help prevent paralysis where none exists currently. By performing these exercises you can maintain flexibility and muscle tone, while you promote the vital flow of blood and lymph to the affected areas. Additionally, most people will experience definite improvement in their total flexibility.

Perform these exercises only if you are unable to do the active exercises described in the other chapters, but return to the others as soon as you can, because they do provide better overall conditioning. If you want a broader workout for a particular joint or muscle group, check the chart on pages 144–49 to see which exercises in the active series have been marked 'Passive'. You can approximate these particular exercises by using your unaffected limb to move or press against the other, just as we illustrate in this chapter.

Exercises 52 to 70 deal with flexibility and require some joint movement. Exercises 71 to 88 are isometric strengtheners that do not require the active movement of a painful joint. Unfortunately, because they do require the ability to contract muscles, people who are paralysed will not be able to perform some of them.

If your joints are stationary, muscle tone and strength are quickly lost when isometric exercises are discontinued. To counter this quick loss of conditioning, the exercises must be done as frequently as possible until more active exercises can be resumed. We recommend that the isometric workout be performed at least daily, and even twice a day if you are up to it.

Before you begin your workout we urge you to speak frankly with your doctor to gain a realistic understanding of just how much strength and movement you can expect to develop, and whether you should ignore some discomfort in order to reach the upper ranges of your goal. *Unless you are specifically instructed to work through that discomfort or pain, you must stop to avoid causing more, and perhaps even permanent, damage to that part of your body.*

PASSIVE EXERCISES FOR FLEXIBILITY

52. The Winner

Sit comfortably and grasp the wrist of your affected arm with your opposite hand, palms down. Raise both arms directly overhead, or as high as you can. Hold for a count of three, and return to the starting position. Repeat.

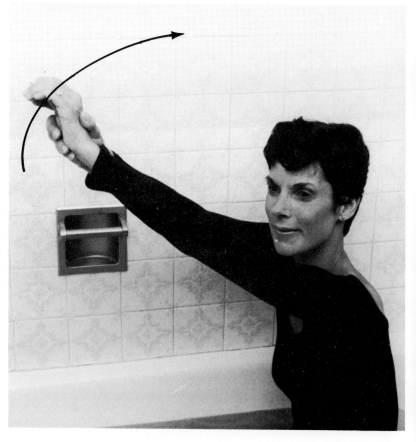

☐ Shoulders/Upper Arms/Passive

53. Horizontal Wrist Circles

Grasp the wrist of your affected arm with your other hand, both palms down. Bring the affected wrist across your body as far as you can, keeping it as low to the floor as possible. Circle it outwards until you touch the side of the bath, then bend your elbow and continue the circle inwards near your body. Repeat. Reverse and circle. Your movements must be slow and controlled. Hold your back straight throughout this exercise.

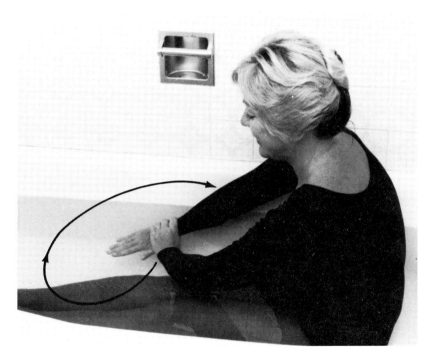

☐ Shoulders/Upper Arms/Elbows/Passive

54. Vertical Wrist Circles

Hold the affected wrist with your other hand. Move both arms to the right as far as possible. Circle your arms up and to the left over your head, then back down to the starting position. Repeat. Reverse the circle, keeping your arms low as they move to the left. Repeat.

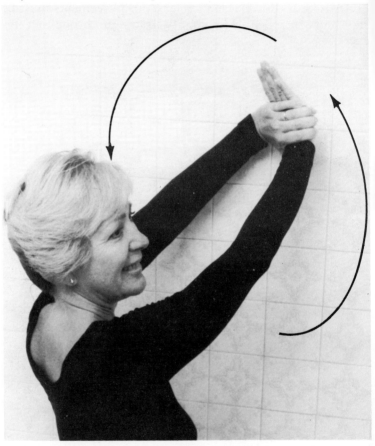

☐ Shoulders/Torso/Upper Back/Passive

55. Shoulder Touch

Sit comfortably and grasp the wrist of the affected arm with your opposite hand. Lift your affected hand straight up until it contacts its shoulder. Your affected elbow will remain at your waist throughout the exercise. Relax and repeat.

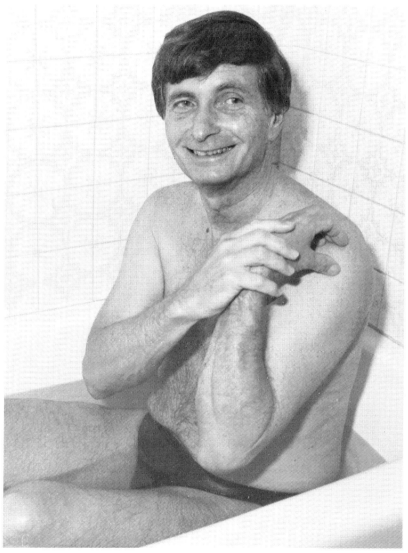

☐ Elbows/Passive

56. Assisted Rotating Palms

Sit comfortably and grasp the palm and back of your affected hand with your good hand. Use your good hand to rotate the other palm up, and then back down again. Repeat.

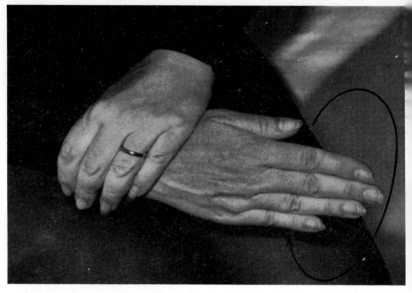

☐ Elbows/Passive

57. Finger Spread

Rest your affected hand palm-up on your lap. Use the other hand gently to spread and circle each finger individually, beginning with the little finger. Progress towards the index finger, then work back down again, this time circling each finger in the other direction. Repeat.

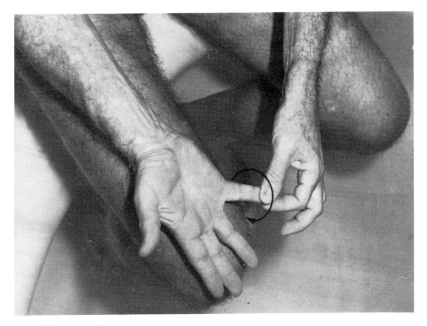

☐Fingers/Passive

58. Finger Backbends

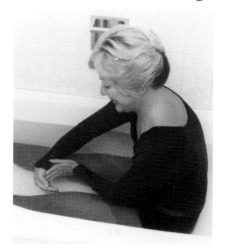

Rest your affected arm comfortably on its thigh as you use the palm and fingers of your other hand slowly and gently to bend the affected fingers backwards. Your wrist will bend also. Relax and repeat.

☐ Fingers/Wrists/Passive

59. Assisted Finger Curls

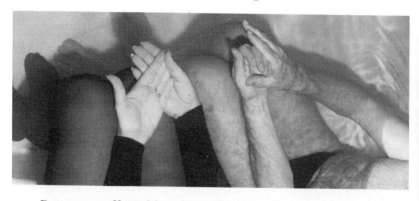

Rest your affected hand on your lap with your extended fingers together. Use your other hand slowly and gently to curl all your fingers into your palm, and then return them to the extended position. Repeat. You may also curl each finger and your thumb separately.

☐ Hands/Fingers/Passive

60. Thumb Circles

Rest your affected hand on your lap with your palm up and your fingers extended comfortably. Use your other hand slowly and gently to move your thumb in a broad circle. Repeat. Reverse the circle and repeat.

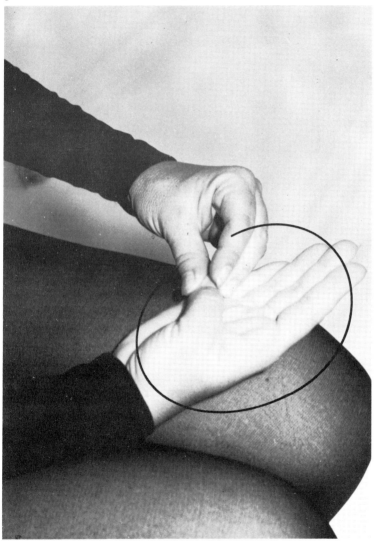

☐ Hands/Fingers/Passive

61. Top-Bends

Rest your comfortably cupped affected hand on top of your good hand, which has been positioned on your lap. Use your good thumb to curl the other backwards and forwards as far as you can without pain. Concentrate the motion at the top joint of the affected thumb, not the joint connecting the thumb to your hand. Repeat.

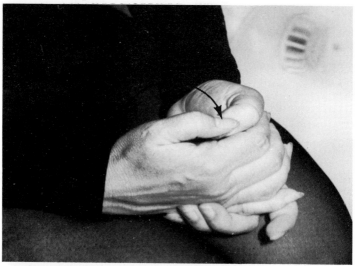

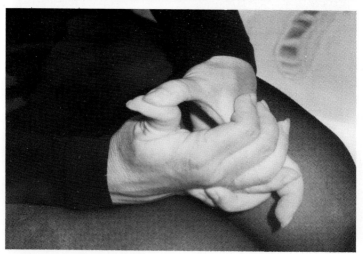

☐ Hands/Fingers/Passive

62. Thumb Up and Over

Rest your affected hand on your lap with your palm up and your fingers extended comfortably. Use your other hand slowly and gently to lift your thumb up and across your palm until it touches the base of your little finger. Return it to the starting position and repeat.

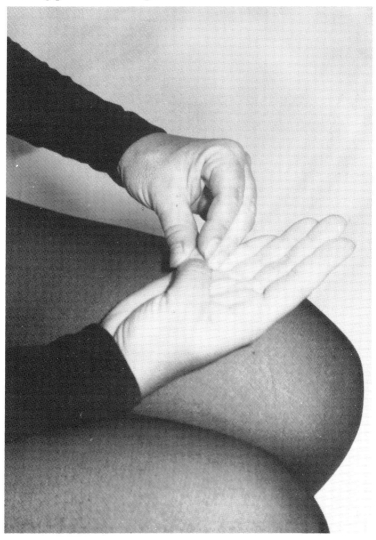

☐ Hands/Fingers/Passive

63. Assisted Leg Lift

Lean back and position your arms on either side of the bath ledge to brace yourself securely. Slip the top of your unaffected foot underneath either your heel or the calf of your affected leg and lift both legs as high as you can. Hold for a count of three, and gently return your feet to the bottom. Rest and repeat. For more strengthening of your abdominal muscles you may sit up straight as you lift your legs.

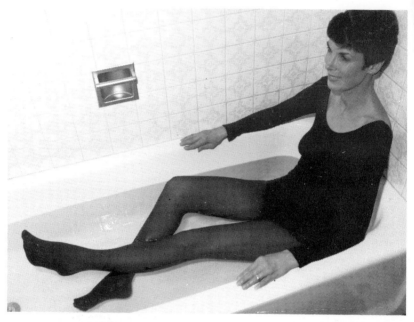

☐ Abdomen/Hips/Passive

CAUTION: *Discontinue this exercise if you experience any discomfort in your back.*

64. Foot Slide

Sit straight with your legs extended. Place one hand on the shin of your affected leg and the other under the thigh. Gently lift your knee towards your chest. Your foot will slide along the bottom of the bath. You may press one hand against your shin to help your knee bend more. Return to the starting position and repeat.

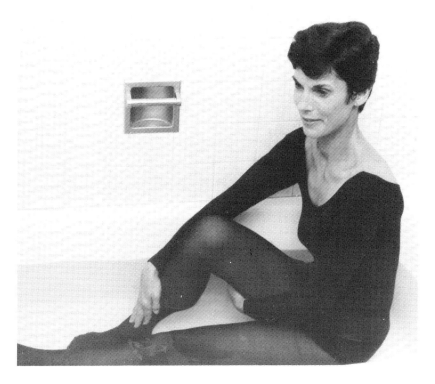

☐ Knees/Hips/Passive

CAUTION: *Discontinue this exercise if you experience any discomfort in your back.*

People with knee replacements or pins must not force the affected leg farther than it can move naturally when supported under the upper part of the leg.

65. Assisted Push and Pull

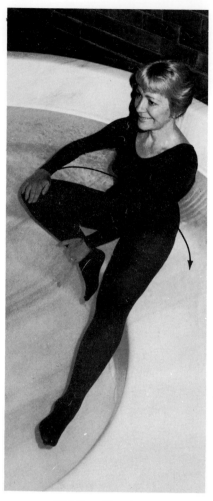

Bend your affected leg comfortably. Grasp your ankle with the opposite hand and use the hand on the same side to push your knee sideways gently, away from the centre of your body. It is OK to let your foot roll on to its outer edge. Now rotate the knee towards the other leg as far as you can. Your foot may roll on to its inner edge. Repeat.

☐ Hips/Passive

CAUTION: *People with hip replacements or pins must not move the foot of the affected leg past the midpoint of their bodies.*

66. One Foot Helps the Other

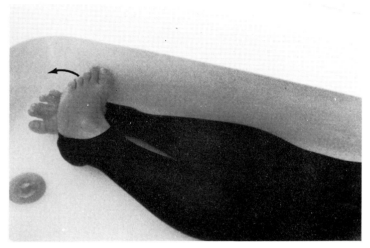

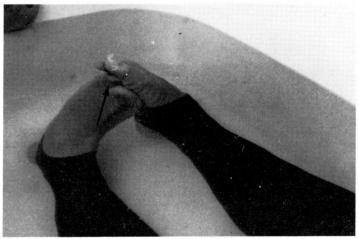

Extend your affected leg and relax your ankle completely. Your foot will curve inwards naturally and your heel will rest on the floor of the tub. Place the sole of the other foot on top of the affected foot, just beneath the place where your toes join your foot. Press downwards gently and release slowly. Now place the top of the other foot beneath the arch of the affected one and gently push it up until the toes of the affected foot point at the ceiling. Release slowly and repeat the sequence.

☐ Ankles/Passive

67. Toe Bends

Extend your affected leg and relax your ankle completely.
Your foot will curve inwards naturally and your heel will rest
on the floor of the bath. Place the sole of the other foot on top
of the affected toes. Press downwards gently to curl your toes.
Release. Now put the top of the other foot beneath the toes of
the affected one and use it to push the affected toes up and
backwards gently as far as they will move. Release slowly and
repeat the sequence.

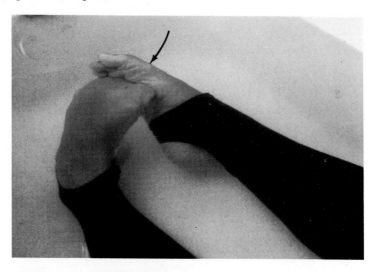

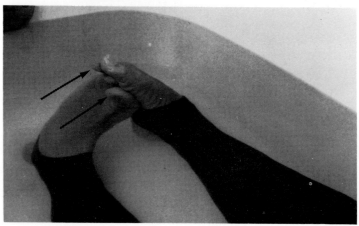

☐ Ankles/Toes/Passive

68. Toe Bends by Hand

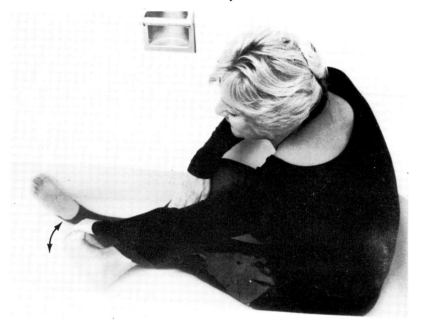

Bend the knee of your affected leg and place it over your extended good leg. Grasp your affected toes with the opposite hand and gently bend them backwards and forwards. Repeat.

☐ Toes/Passive

69. Foot-Waving by Hand

Sit up straight and extend your good leg forward. Place the calf of your affected leg over it as far up towards your body as you can with comfort. Grasp the ball of your foot with the hand on the unaffected side of your body and use it to wave your foot up and down. It is OK to bend forward to reach your foot, if necessary. Repeat.

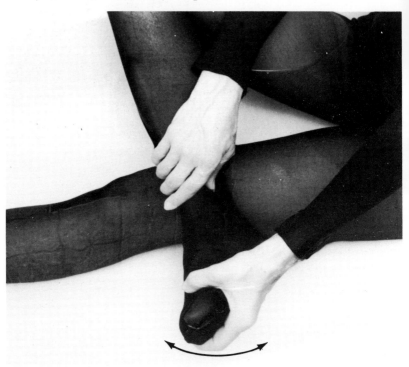

☐ Ankles/Toes/Passive

70. Foot Circles by Hand

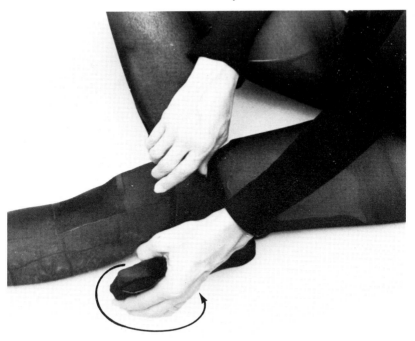

Sit up straight and extend your good leg forward. Place the calf of your affected leg over it as far up towards your body as you can with comfort. Grasp the ball of your foot with the hand on the unaffected side of your body and use it to move the foot in a smooth circle. Repeat. You will feel motion in your ankle. It is OK to bend forward to reach your foot, if necessary. Reverse the circle and repeat.

☐ Torso/Ankles/Passive

ISOMETRICS FOR STRENGTHENING

71. Waist Press

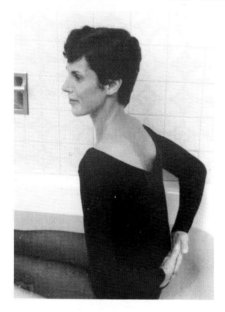

With your hands behind your back, palms facing away from your body and your elbows comfortably bent, place your right hand over your left as you press both hands into the small of your back and release. Repeat. Reverse the position of your hands and repeat.

☐ Upper Arms/Lower Arms/Hands

72. Tummy Flatteners

Sit up straight, take a deep breath, and draw in your stomach and abdominal muscles as tightly as you can. Keep them tense as you slowly count aloud to ten. Exhale, relax completely, and repeat.

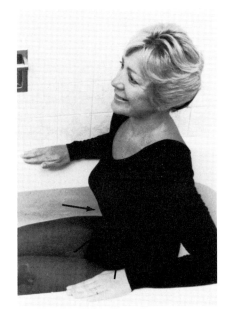

☐ Torso/Abdomen

73. Forehead Flattener

Place the back of your right hand in your left palm and use it to press the back of your left hand to your forehead. Elbows are extended to the side with the tips pointed back as far as possible. Hold for a count of six. Relax and repeat.

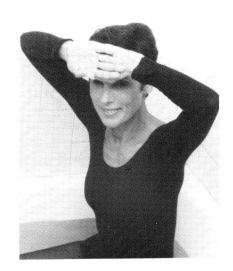

☐ Neck/Upper Arms/Lower Arms/Hands

74. Chin Thrust

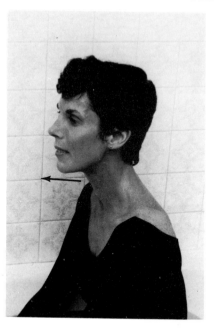

Sit up straight and thrust your head forward. Keep your chin level, and don't clench your teeth. Hold for a count of six, and relax. Repeat.

☐ Neck

75. Elbow to Elbow

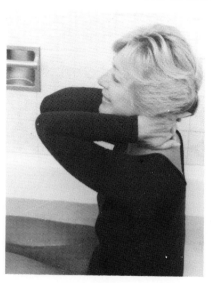

Gently interlace your fingers behind your neck, elbows forward. You may put the fingers of one hand on top of the fingers of the other, if you wish. Push your head backwards as you try to touch elbows, if possible. Relax and repeat.

☐ Neck/Lower Arms/ Hands/Fingers

76. Prayer Position

Tuck your elbows into your sides at the waist and extend your lower arms horizontally. Bring your palms together, wrists straight and fingers extended. Press palms against each other and hold for a count of six. Relax and repeat.

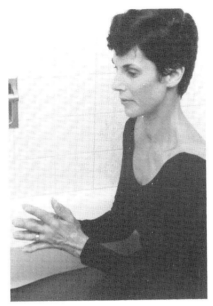

☐ Upper Arms/Lower Arms/Hands

77. Extended Prayer Position

Extend your straight arms directly in front of your body, about waist high. Press your palms together, wrists straight and fingers extended. Hold for a count of six. Relax and repeat.

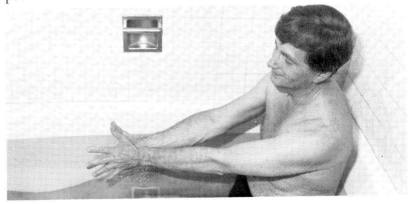

☐ Upper Arms/Lower Arms/Hands

78. Fist-over-Fist Press

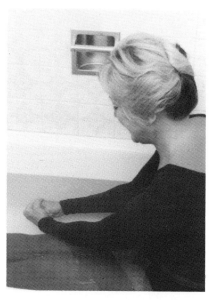

Close your left hand over your right fist, palms towards your chest, wrists as straight as possible. Move your elbows slightly in front of your body but in line with your shoulders. Press your hands into one another and hold for a count of six. Relax and repeat. Reverse the position of your hands and repeat.

☐ Upper Arms/Lower Arms/Hands

79. Finger Press

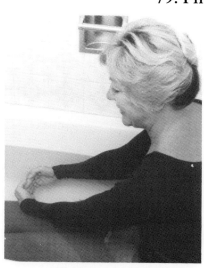

Close your left hand over the bent fingers of your right hand, palms towards your chest, wrists as straight as possible. Move your elbows slightly in front of your body but in line with your shoulders. Press the fingers of your right hand into your left palm, as if trying to straighten them. Hold for a count of six. Relax and repeat. Reverse the position of your hands and repeat.

☐ Upper Arms/Lower Arms/Hands/Fingers

80. Thigh Press

Place your palms midway up the front of each thigh, wrists slightly cocked, fingers extended. Press downwards and hold for a count of six. Relax and repeat.

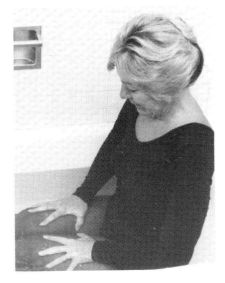

☐ Upper Arms/Lower Arms/Hands/Fingers

81. Knee/Palm Press

Place your hands on your knees and press down as you push up with your knees. Hold in your abdominal muscles as you press down, but don't forget to breathe. Hold for a count of six. Relax and repeat.

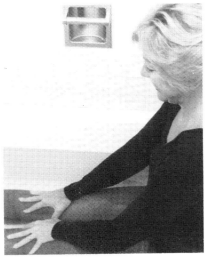

☐ Upper Arms/Lower Arms/Hands/Fingers/Abdomen/ Upper Legs

82. Criss-Crossed Wrists

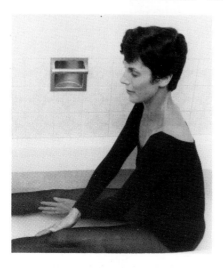

Spread your legs comfortably and cross your wrists, so that your right palm rests against the inside of your left thigh and your left palm is against the inside of your right thigh. Press your palms into your thighs as you resist the pressure with your thigh muscles. Hold for a count of six. Relax and repeat.

☐ Upper Arms/Lower Arms/Hands/Upper Legs

83. Criss-Crossed Forearms

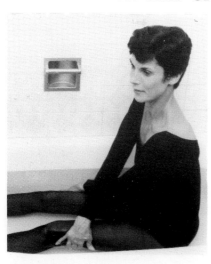

Cross your forearms and grasp the outside of your left thigh with your right hand and the outside of your right thigh with your left hand, several inches above each knee. Press inwards with your palms and outwards with your thighs. Hold for a count of six. Relax and repeat.

☐ Upper Arms/Lower Arms/Hands/Upper Legs

The following exercises require two half-gallon or two 2-litre plastic bottles or jugs (lemonade-bottles work nicely) and an ordinary facecloth. One bottle will always be capped and empty. The other can be capped and filled with bathwater. Just submerge the bottle to fill it, and then empty the water back into the bath when you have finished. These exercises should be omitted if preparing or using the items causes discomfort.

84. Tug-of-War

With your elbows straight and hands submerged, palms down, grasp a facecloth securely with your hands and pull it taut horizontally. Hold for a count of six. Relax and repeat. Now pull it taut vertically, positioning your right hand higher than your left. Keep both hands submerged, if possible. Hold for a count of six. Relax and repeat, this time with your left hand higher than your right. Repeat.

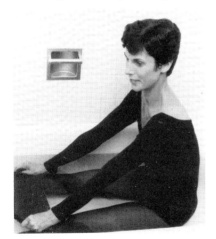 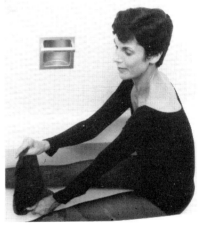

☐ Upper Arms/Lower Arms/Fingers

CAUTION: *Omit this exercise if grasping the cloth causes pain to fingers or hands.*

85. Toe Tug-of-War

Grasp a facecloth as securely as you can using only the toes of each foot. It may take a while to do this adequately, but that is part of the exercise. Pull the cloth horizontally until each side is taut. Hold for a count of six. Relax and repeat. Now simultaneously pull the cloth up with the toes of your right foot and down with the toes of the left. Hold for a count of six. Relax, then repeat with the left foot up and the right down. Try to keep your feet submerged at all times.

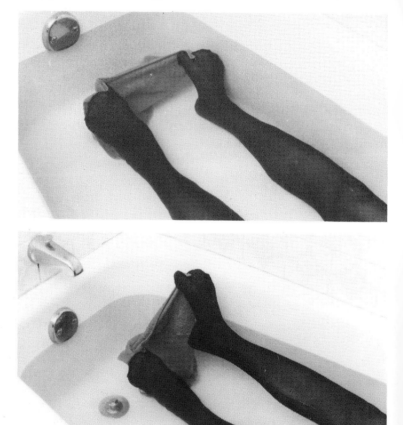

☐ Abdomen/Upper Legs/Lower Legs/Toes

CAUTION: *Omit this exercise if grasping the cloth causes pain or cramping in your toes, feet or legs.*

86. Bottle Bounce

Put your palms on either side of a capped empty 2-litre plastic bottle positioned horizontally between your outspread knees. Keep your elbows straight as you press down very slowly until the bottle just touches the bottom of the bath. Allow it to return gently to the top of the water. Repeat, using slow, controlled movements. Repeat, using just one hand. Switch to the other hand and repeat.

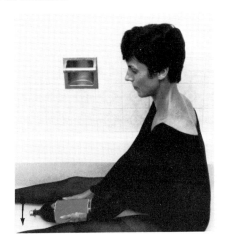

☐ Upper Arms/Lower Arms/Hands

87. Bottle Press

Extend your arms and put your palms on either side of a full 2-litre plastic bottle held just under the top of the water. Squeeze and hold for a count of six. Relax and repeat. Now straighten your elbows and continue to squeeze and relax. Repeat.

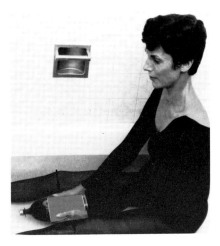

☐ Upper Arms/Lower Arms/Hands

88. Foot Press

Place the filled 2-litre plastic bottle between the soles of your feet and press. Your knees may be bent or extended. Hold for a count of six. Relax and repeat.

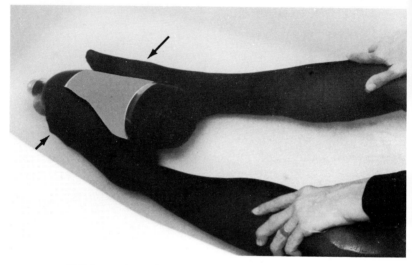

☐ Upper Legs/Lower Legs/Feet

6

Aerobic Exercises

Aerobic exercises condition your heart and belong in any well-rounded exercise regimen. However, some of these exercises may be too difficult for you at the beginning of your programme, and you may find that you must work into them gradually. Cut back immediately on the number of repetitions or the vigour with which you perform them if you find your pulse rate elevated beyond the limits recommended by your doctor or in the table on page 141.

A general guideline for performing these aerobic exercises in comfortably warm water is about fifteen or twenty minutes at least three times a week. However, your doctor should be the person to instruct you on how long to sustain the aerobic portion of your exercises, taking into account the total amount of exercising you do from the other chapters in this book and the rate at which you perform them. Bear in mind that water temperature plays a large part in the determination of the amount of aerobic exercise time you allow. *Follow your doctor's recommendations explicitly.*

Remember, too, that any exercise that requires you to circle or swing your arms or legs can have considerable aerobic value if done rapidly. You may want to include some of the exercises from Chapter 4 in the aerobic portion of your workout, particularly those that feel as though they 'hit' your trouble spots.

89. Reach for the Gold

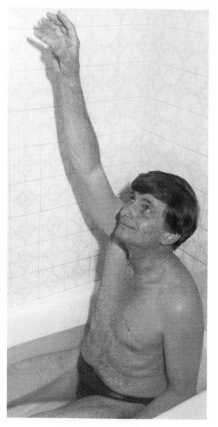

Sit upright and imagine that the branches of a tree full of solid-gold apples are hanging directly overhead. Reach up with your open hand, grasp a golden apple, and pull your closed fist all the way down to your side, as if putting it into the side-pocket of your trousers. Repeat, alternating right and left hands.

☐ Shoulders/Elbows/Hands/Fingers/Torso/Waist/ Aerobic

90. Crossovers

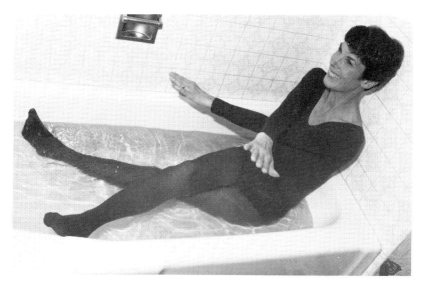

Balance yourself carefully as you spread your straight arms to the side, as wide as possible. At the same time spread and lift your slightly bent legs off the bottom of the bath at least several inches, or higher if you can. Now swing your arms and legs across your body as far as you can and then back to the original spread position. Repeat the action as smoothly and quickly as you can.

☐ Shoulders/Upper Arms/Abdomen/Hips/Upper Legs/ Aerobic

CAUTION: *People with shoulder or hip replacements or pins must not move their affected hands or feet past the midpoint of their bodies.*

91. Swing Your Elbows

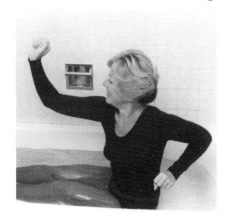

Sit upright and slide forward far enough so that you can swing your elbows behind you without hitting the back of the bath. With each hand in a loosely closed fist, cock each elbow so that forearms and upper arms are at a 90° angle to one another, right arm to the front and left arm behind. Raise both elbows out of the water. Try to get your right elbow all the way up to eye level and the left as high as your shoulder, but don't be discouraged if neither moves quite this far. Reverse your arm positions. Repeat, performing the movement as vigorously as possible, even though you splash a little in the process.

☐ Shoulders/Upper Back/Torso/Elbows/Aerobic

92. Breaststroke Triangle

Lean forward slightly, arms outstretched, hands just under the top of the water with their backs touching. Your thumbs point downwards and your fingers are together and slightly cupped. Bend your elbows as you draw your hands apart and back until your thumbs rest lightly on each hip. Draw your hands together at your waist, palms facing one another, thumbs up, as if you are saying a prayer. Now straighten your elbows until your arms are fully extended just under the top of the water. The complete motion traces a skinny triangle. Rotate your wrists so that your thumbs again point downwards, and repeat.

Now reverse the motion. Begin by bending your elbows and turning your palms forward at your hips. Straighten your elbows as you push the water forward, allowing your palms to come together when your arms are fully extended. While your palms are still touching, return your hands to your body, stopping when both wrists come to rest gently at the centre of your abdomen. Move both hands back to your hips. Repeat.

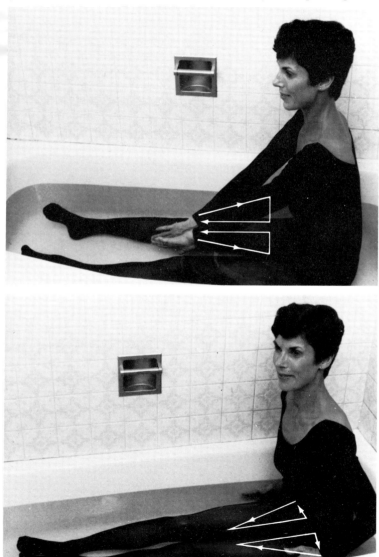

☐ Shoulders/Arms/Elbows/Wrists/Aerobic

93. Foot Drag

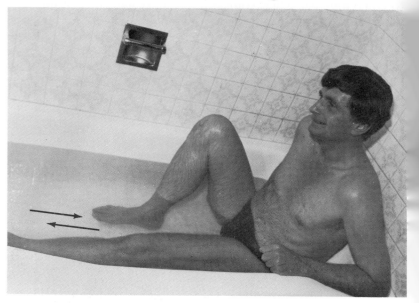

Sit up straight with your legs extended. Brace yourself firmly. Bend your right knee and drag your right foot towards your body until it is as close as you can get it. Be sure your foot is in contact with the bottom of the bath at all times. Straighten your right knee while you simultaneously bend your left knee and drag your left foot on the bottom of the bath until it is close to your body. Repeat and speed up the motion as much as possible.

☐ Hips/Knees/Aerobic

94. Tricycle

Slouch down and brace yourself firmly. Your pelvis should be thrust as far forward and upward as possible. Extend your right leg forward as you lift your bent left knee upward. Your knee, lower leg and toes may break the waterline. Your lower leg will be parallel to the bottom of the bath. Point your toes to the ceiling at all times. Now alternate your leg position. Your feet will make small circles, just as if you are riding a child's tricycle, as your knees alternately bend and straighten. Your rhythm must be smooth, steady and moderately rapid.

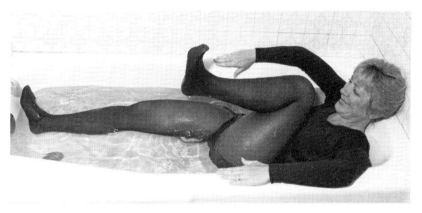

☐ Abdomen/Hips/Upper Legs/Knees/Lower Legs/ Ankles/Aerobic

CAUTION: *Discontinue this exercise if you experience any discomfort in your back.*

95. Arm and Leg Co-ordination

Sit upright and slide far enough forward so that you can swing your elbows behind you without hitting the back of the bath. Bend your left elbow and touch your left hand to your rib-cage. Your right arm is extended straight forward, hand open. Simultaneously extend your right leg forward, keeping it as straight as you can, while your left knee is drawn up as close to your chin as possible. Now reverse the positions of your arms and legs so that your left arm and left leg are extended and your right arm and right leg are bent. Repeat, making the motion as rhythmic and rapid as possible.

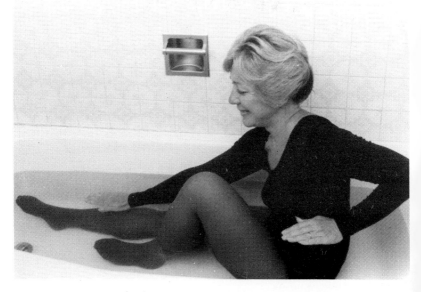

☐ Shoulders/Upper Arms/Lower Arms/Elbows/Wrists/ Hands/Hips/Upper Legs/Knees/Ankles/Co-ordination/ Aerobic

7

Exercises for Spa and Hot Tub Only

The exercises in this chapter have been created specifically for a spa workout because of the broad side-to-side movements that are simply impossible in a conventional bathtub. However, all the exercises in the other chapters are easily adapted to spa or hot tub and should become an integral part of your exercise programme.

Be sure to maintain your balance by bracing yourself with your hands and arms whenever necessary, using any position that you find comfortable.

To simplify the illustration of certain multimovement exercises we have photographed several models together in the spa. 'Read' these pictures from left to right to understand the proper sequence of movements.

96. Flutter Kick

Lean back and brace yourself firmly against the back of the spa. Extend your legs, knees slightly flexed but not bent at a sharp angle. Toes point upwards, not forwards. Alternately move each leg up and down as far as possible with a smooth steady rhythm. All motion comes from your hips, not from your knees. Do not draw your knees towards your face.

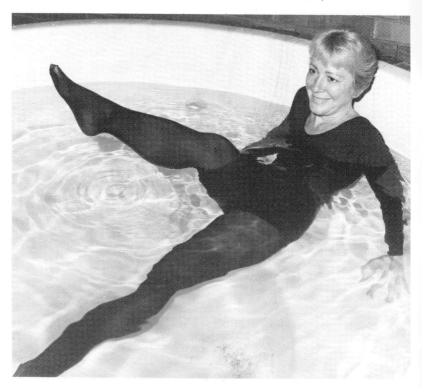

☐ Abdomen/Upper Legs/Hips

97. Great Big Circles

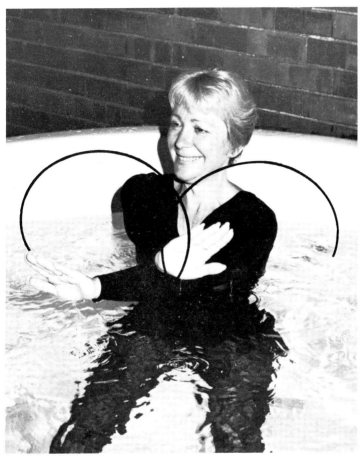

Sit comfortably and raise your straight arms to the side, as you circle them upwards towards each other and then down past the front of your body. You may cross them in order to make your circles larger. Your arms should make the widest circle possible. Repeat. Now, reverse the direction of the swing so that your arms rise as they move to the centre of your body and away from each other and lower as they move behind you. Repeat.

☐ Shoulders/Torso/Upper Back/Passive

CAUTION: *People with shoulder replacements or pins must not move the affected arm past the midpoint of their bodies.*

119

98. Ballet Bend

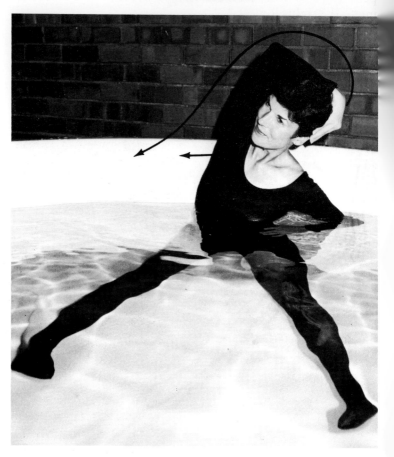

Sit straight, legs extended and comfortably spread. Place your left hand on the side of your waist. Your right arm is extended to the side in line with your left shoulder, palm up. Raise your straight right arm overhead. Your upper arm should rest against your right ear if possible. Bend your torso to the left as you bend and curl your right elbow over the top of your head, as if attempting to touch your left earlobe with your fingers. Keep both buttocks firmly on the tub floor at all times. The movement is smooth and controlled. Do not bounce sideways in an attempt to increase the waist bend. Return to the upright position with your right arm again extended to the side. Repeat. Reverse sides, this time raising your left arm and bending to the right. Repeat.

☐ Shoulders/Elbows/Wrists/Torso/Lower Back

CAUTION: *Discontinue this exercise if you experience any discomfort in your back.*

99. Body Twists

Sit up with your legs straight and comfortably spread. Interlock your fingers, or cup one hand in the other if that is more comfortable. Raise and extend your arms until they are parallel to the floor. Swing them to the right and then to the left as far as you can. Make just one smooth arc in each direction. Your buttocks must be firmly on the spa bottom at all times. Repeat.

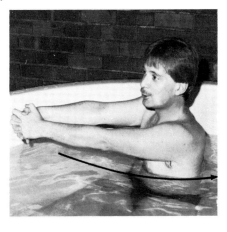

☐ Shoulders/Torso/Lower Back

CAUTION: *People with low-back pain must keep their knees slightly bent during this exercise. If you experience pain in your back while doing this exercise, stop immediately but continue with the remainder of the programme. At the next exercise session bend or stretch only to the point where you do not feel any pain, or omit the exercise entirely.*

100. Crazy Legs

Sit up straight and extend both feet forward, toes pointed up and ankles touching. Bend and spread your knees while you turn your feet outwards until your soles are pressed together and the outer edge of each foot rests on the spa bottom. Slide your feet towards your body, as close as possible. Your knees should be as near to the floor as you can get them, but do not press them downward with your hands. Now lift your left knee up, as if to touch the tip of your left shoulder but do not bring your shoulder forward. Your foot will leave the spa bottom. Return to the spread position. Repeat, lifting your right knee to your right shoulder. Return to the spread position and then slide both feet forward to the original extended-leg position. Repeat.

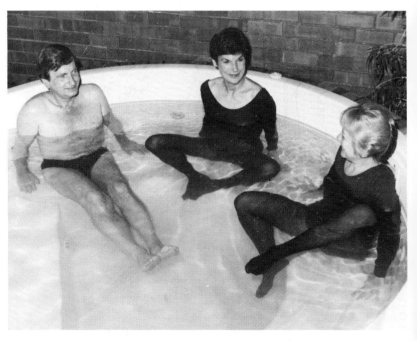

☐ Abdomen/Hips/Knees

101. Single-Leg Triangles

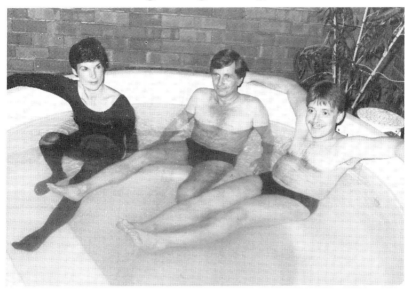

Slide your right foot towards your body until your knee is as close to your chin as you can get it. Your left leg is positioned at the front of your body, either comfortably outstretched, or bent if you prefer. Straighten your right leg completely as you thrust it as far to the right as you can. Your toes point to the ceiling. Now swing your straight right leg to the front as you simultaneously straighten your left leg forwards and upwards until your ankles touch. The toes of both feet now point to the ceiling, breaking the waterline if possible. Hold for a count of three. Rest for a count of one, and repeat. All movements are rapid but smooth. Repeat the sequence with your left leg.

☐ Abdomen/Hips/Knees/Upper Legs

102. Reverse Single-Leg Triangles

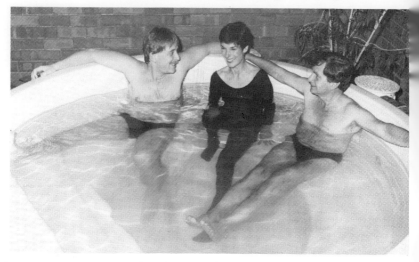

Stretch your straight right leg as far as you can to the right. Your left leg is positioned at the front of your body, either comfortably outstretched, or bent if you prefer. Now bend your right knee and draw it towards you until your foot points forward and is as close to your body as is comfortable. Thrust both legs forward and upward simultaneously, ankles together and toes pointed towards the ceiling. Your toes should break the waterline if possible. Hold for a count of three. Rest for a count of one, and repeat. Repeat the sequence with your left leg.

☐ Abdomen/Hips/Knees/Upper Legs

103. Froggie Kick

This variation of Single-Leg Triangles (exercise 101) uses both legs simultaneously. Sit up and extend both legs to the front, ankles together, toes pointing to the ceiling. Slide both feet towards you by bending your knees and bringing them as close to your chest as possible. You may raise your feet if necessary. Now straighten both legs completely as you thrust them sideways as far as you can, toes again pointing to the ceiling. Return your straight legs to the starting position. Hold for a count of three. Rest for a count of one, and repeat. The motion is done smoothly and as rapidly as possible, but be sure to rest between each repetition.

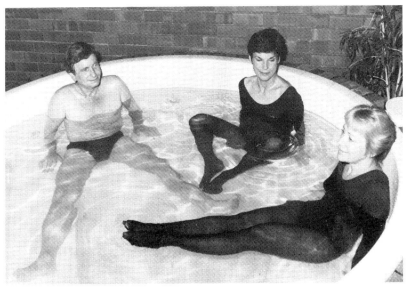

☐ Abdomen/Hips/Knees/Upper Legs

104. Reverse Froggie Kick

This variation of the Reverse Single-Leg Triangle (exercise 102) uses both legs simultaneously. Sit up straight and extend both legs to the front, ankles together, toes pointing to the ceiling. Begin by sliding each leg as far as you can to its respective side. Now bend both knees and bring them as close to your chest as possible. Straighten your legs and return them to the starting position. Rest for a count of one, and repeat.

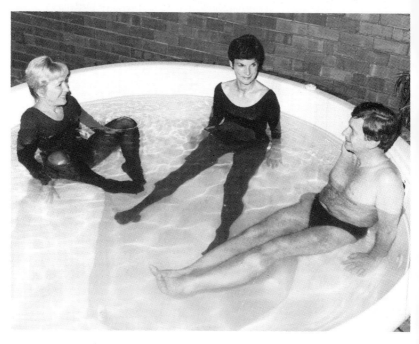

☐ Abdomen/Hips/Knees/Upper Legs

105. Elementary Backstroke

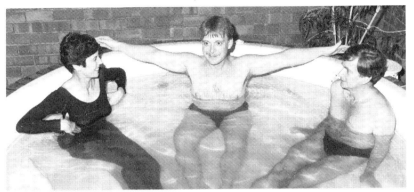

Bend and raise your elbows to shoulder height, while you run your fingers up each side of your torso until they reach your armpits. Now extend your arms to each side, elbows and hands at shoulder level. Swing both arms straight down to your sides until your palms rest on the bottom of the spa.

☐ Shoulders/Elbows/Wrists/Upper Arms/Lower Arms

106. Elementary Backstroke with Kick

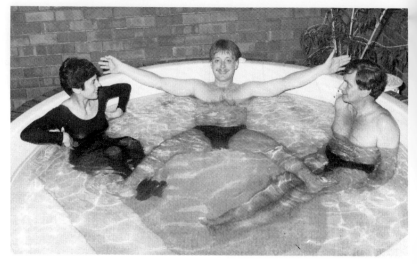

This variation of the Elementary Backstroke (exercise 105) combines its movements with those of a kick. Be sure you are firmly braced so you don't lose your balance. Bend your knees and elbows simultaneously, extend them to the side at the same time, and then return both to the resting position, hands at your sides and legs extended. Rest and repeat.

☐   Shoulders/Elbows/Wrists/Abdomen/Hips/Knees/ Upper Arms/Lower Arms/Upper Legs/Co-ordination

8

Massage

Gentle massage of painful body areas, no matter how well performed and no matter how much better you feel afterwards, cannot replace a well-designed exercise regimen. Massage should be viewed as a helpful, relaxing adjunct to exercise that has the additional benefit of helping to promote good blood circulation. Massage can be enjoyed before you begin your exercise session to help loosen joints and muscles, during the session to relieve momentary muscle cramping, or after you have finished as a bit of constructive pampering for sore muscles and joints. We focus on arms, legs and feet in this section, as these are the places where acute cramping most often occurs.

Keep in mind that stressing any part of your body to the point of pain during your regular exercise programme must be avoided unless your doctor recommends otherwise. If you feel strongly in need of a massage after you have finished exercising but really didn't need it before you began, you are probably doing too much and should cut back temporarily on the number of repetitions of each exercise that involves the problem area, or should do those exercises less vigorously.

A gently performed massage in a pleasantly warm bath, especially with aching muscles or joints submerged, is more effective than the same massage done out of water, even when you use expensive friction-reducing creams or lotions.

We suggest that you stabilize yourself by bracing your knees or forearms against the bath to prevent slipping, whenever possible. Bending your knees slightly when your legs are extended so that your heels can rest on the bottom of the bath is better than thrusting them out directly in front of you. This position also makes it easier to reach your lower calf, foot and toes. Bending the knees so much that the foot rests flat on the bottom of the bath is uncomfortable for some people. They should not bend their legs that much.

107. Hand Massage

Rest your relaxed left arm on your lap and imagine that you are using your right hand to pull on and smooth a tight left glove. Beginning with your thumb, gently smooth each finger in turn. Continue rubbing your fingers down past the top of your hand in a straight line to your wrist. Repeat. Change hands and repeat.

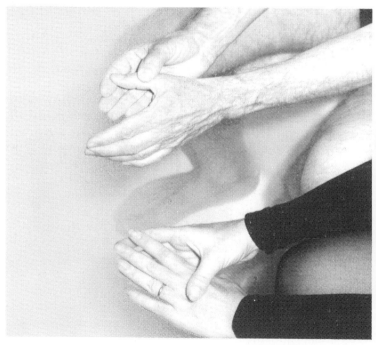

☐ Hands/Fingers

108. Elbow Massage

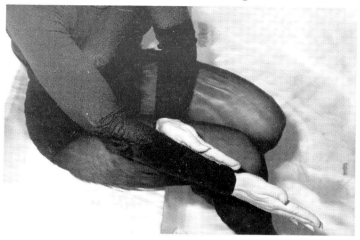

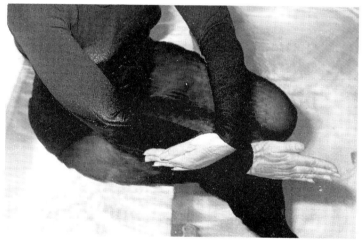

Rub your left palm firmly up the inside of your right forearm, beginning at the fingertips of your right hand. Continue rubbing across your elbow and back down to your hand. Repeat. Now, begin at the outside of your hand and move up your forearm to your elbow and back down to your hand. Repeat the sequence with your right palm against your left arm.

☐ Elbows/Lower Arms/Hands

CAUTION: *Don't apply pressure with your fingertips because you can hurt the small joints.*

109. Elbow-to-Shoulder Massage

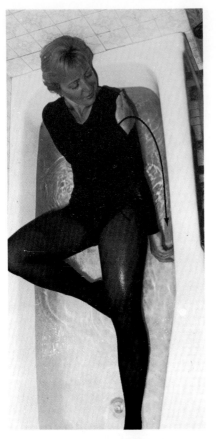

Lean back and slide down so that your shoulders are submerged as far as is comfortable. Rub your right palm firmly on your left upper arm, beginning at the inside elbow and working up and over the shoulder and down the outside of your forearm, crossing the elbow joint. Repeat. Now repeat, using your left palm on your right arm.

☐ Shoulders/Upper Arms/Elbows

CAUTION: *Don't apply pressure with your fingertips because you can hurt the small joints.*

110. Finger Walking

With your shoulders still sub-merged, walk the fingers of your right hand rapidly but gently up and down your left arm, beginning at the inside of your left wrist, past the el-bow, up and over the shoulder, and back down the outside of your arm to the wrist. Repeat. Reverse the exercise and begin at your outer wrist and work up, in-wards, and down. Repeat, using your left hand to mass-age your right arm.

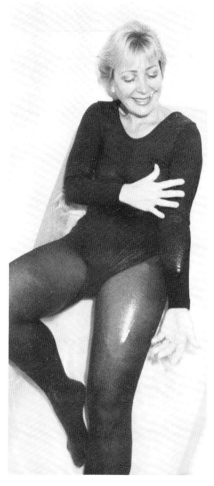

☐ Shoulders/Upper Arms/Elbows/Lower Arms/Fingers

CAUTION: *Discontinue massage if the light pressure exerted on your fingers becomes painful.*

111. Upper-Leg Massage

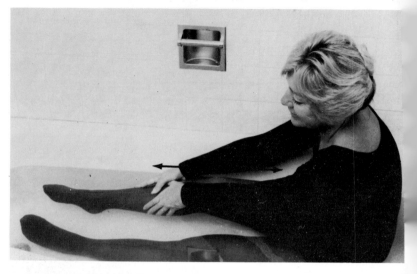

Position the heels of both palms at each side of your right leg below your knee. Your legs may be straight or bent. Rub your open palms firmly upwards to your groin and hip area. Put the pressure on the heels of your hands, not on your fingers. Reverse the motion by stroking gently downwards, until you again reach below the knee. Repeat. Reposition your hands so they rub all areas of your thigh. Repeat the sequence with your left leg.

☐ Upper Legs/Knees

112. Lower–Leg Massage

Lean slightly forward and bend your right leg. Your right sole rests flat on the bottom of the bath. Your left leg is comfortably extended. Position the heels of both hands at the sides of your right knee. Rub your open hands firmly downwards over your knee. Put the pressure on the heels of your hands, not on your fingers. Reverse the motion by stroking gently upwards until you reach the knee again. Reposition your hands so that they will eventually rub all the areas of your lower leg as you continue, but you need not rub your shin bone, which runs down the very front of your lower leg, as bones do not require massage. Repeat the sequence with your left leg.

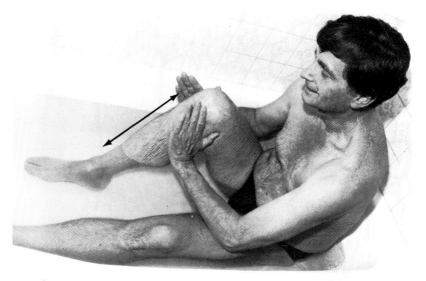

☐ Lower Legs/Knees

113. Full–Leg Massage

Lean forward slightly and place your hands on each side of your right knee. You may bend your knee comfortably as you rub your palms up and down your leg from the knee to the ankle and back, then from the knee to the groin and back. Repeat. Repeat the sequence with your left leg.

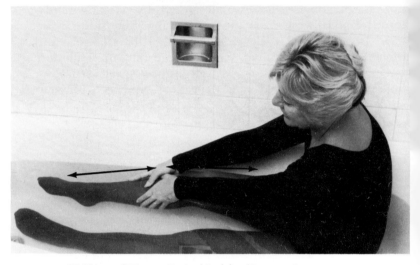

☐ Knees/Upper Legs/Ankles/Lower Legs

114. Finger Jogging

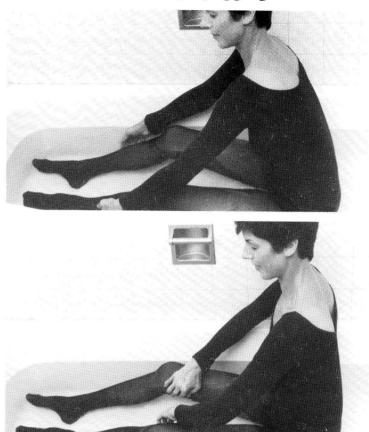

Lean forward with your knees comfortably bent and walk the fingers of both hands rapidly but gently up the outside of your ankles, past your knees, and up to your hips. Cross over the front of your leg to just below your groin and walk your fingers back down the inside of your legs. Repeat, repositioning your fingers slightly each time so that you touch a slightly different area of your legs on each round trip. Reverse direction by beginning the sequence on the inside of your ankles.

☐ Upper Legs/Knees/Lower Legs/Ankles

CAUTION: *Discontinue massage if the light pressure exerted on your fingers becomes painful.*

115. Foot Kneading

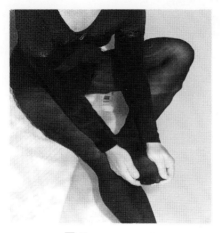

Lean forward slightly and rest the heel of your left foot on your right calf or thigh. Gently knead the ball of your right foot, instep and sole with your palms. Use moderate pressure, alternating with gently squeezing movements. Repeat with the right foot.

☐ Feet

CAUTION: *Don't force your foot upwards if you have pain in your hip, knee or ankle. Discontinue massage if your wrists or fingers and thumbs hurt while applying pressure.*

116. Gentle Circles

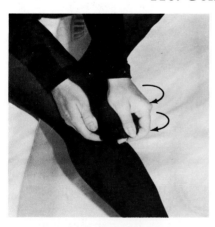

While keeping the heel of your left foot on your right calf or knee, as in the previous exercise, use a gentle circular or elliptical pressure with your palms, beginning with your toes and extending down to the bottom of your left foot and ending under the curve of your heel. Repeat. Change position so that your right foot is resting on your left leg and repeat.

☐ Feet

CAUTION: *Don't force your foot upwards if you feel pain in your hip, knee or ankle. Discontinue massage if your wrists or fingers and thumbs hurt while applying pressure.*

117. Foot-to-Foot Massage

The heel of each foot rests on the bottom of the bath. You will be more comfortable if you bend and spread your knees. Rub the ball of your left foot up and down the length of your right foot. Repeat. Now rub the ball of your right foot up and down the sole of the left. Repeat.

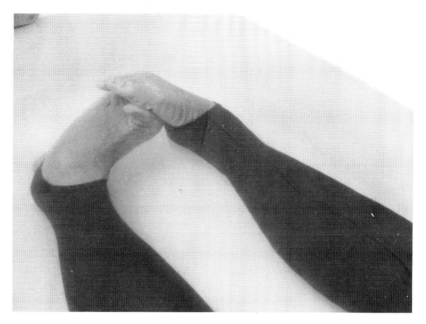

☐ Feet

Appendix A
Finding Your Ideal Exercise Heart (Pulse) Rate

Table 1 lists generally recognized and accepted guidelines for target heartbeat ranges to receive the maximum benefit from the aerobic portion of your exercise session. You must monitor your pulse intermittently during each session, particularly when doing the aerobic workout in Chapter 6. Your doctor's specific recommendations will supersede these guidelines.

Using this table is simple. First count your pulse beats for a full ten seconds. See pages 22-23 for instructions on how to locate your pulse points. Next refer to column 1 to identify your approximate age. Column 2 indicates your ideal minimum and maximum pulse rates for the ten-second monitoring period. This is the range you should strive to sustain while doing the aerobic exercises. Do not exceed the maximum recommended pulse rate without your doctor's specific approval. Column 3 extends then ten-second monitoring period to show the pulse-rate range for one minute.

Recommended heartbeat ranges decrease gradually with advancing age, as you can see. Because our chart is graded in five-year increments we have included the formula that is used to determine heartbeat range (see Appendix B). We also use the mathematical example of a forty-seven-year-old person.

Follow the formula and the example to compute your own individual ideal range.

Table 2 can be used to determine the exact number of times your heart beats each minute, based on the number of pulse beats in a ten-second interval.

Table 1 **Ideal Exercise Heart-Rate Table**

AGE	RECOMMENDED RANGE OF PULSE BEATS FOR 10 SECONDS	PULSE RANGE PER MINUTE
15	24–7	144–64
20	23–7	140–60
25	23–6	137–56
30	22–5	133–52
35	21–4	130–48
40	21–4	126–44
45	20–3	123–40
50	20–3	119–36
55	19–22	116–32
60	19–21	112–28
65	18–21	109–24
70	17–20	105–20
75	17–19	102–16
80	16–19	98–112
85	15–18	95–108
90	15–17	91–104

Table 2 Ten-Second to Per-Minute Heartbeat Conversion Table

NUMBER OF BEATS/10 SEC.	NUMBER OF BEATS/MINUTE
12	72
13	78
14	84
15	90
16	96
17	102
18	108
19	114
20	120
21	126
22	132
23	138
24	144
25	150
26	156
27	162
28	168
29	174

Appendix B
How to Compute Your Exact Exercise Heart Rate

1. Subtract your exact age from the number 220 to find the raw number.

220	Mathematical constant
-47	Age
173	Raw number

2. Multiply the raw number by .7 and round off the result to the nearest whole number. This is the lower exercise limit per minute.

173	Raw number
x .7	
121	Lower limit

3. Divide the lower limit by 6 and round to the nearest whole number to find the lower exercise limit per 10 seconds of monitoring.

20	Minimum beats/
6⟌121	10 sec

4. Multiply the raw number by .8 and round off the result to the nearest whole number. This is the upper exercise limit per minute.

173	Raw number
x .8	
138	Upper limit

5. Divide the upper limit by 6 and round to the nearest whole number to find the upper exercise limit per 10 seconds of monitoring.

23	Maximum beats/
6⟌138	10 secs

Exercise Review Chart

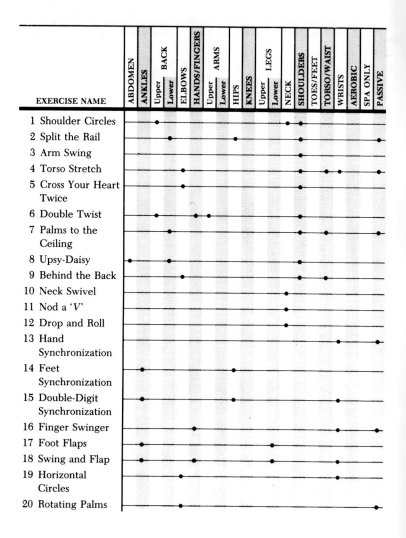

EXERCISE NAME	ABDOMEN	ANKLES	BACK Upper	BACK Lower	ELBOWS	HANDS/FINGERS	ARMS Upper	ARMS Lower	HIPS	KNEES	LEGS Upper	LEGS Lower	NECK	SHOULDERS	TOES/FEET	TORSO/WAIST	WRISTS	AEROBIC	SPA ONLY	PASSIVE
1 Shoulder Circles			•										•	•						
2 Split the Rail				•					•											•
3 Arm Swing			•											•						
4 Torso Stretch				•										•		•				
5 Cross Your Heart Twice				•										•		•				
6 Double Twist				•										•		•				
7 Palms to the Ceiling				•										•			•			
8 Upsy-Daisy	•			•										•						
9 Behind the Back					•									•						
10 Neck Swivel													•							
11 Nod a 'V'													•							
12 Drop and Roll													•							
13 Hand Synchronization																	•			•
14 Feet Synchronization	•								•											
15 Double-Digit Synchronization	•																•			
16 Finger Swinger						•														•
17 Foot Flaps	•																			
18 Swing and Flap	•					•										•				
19 Horizontal Circles						•											•			
20 Rotating Palms		•																		•

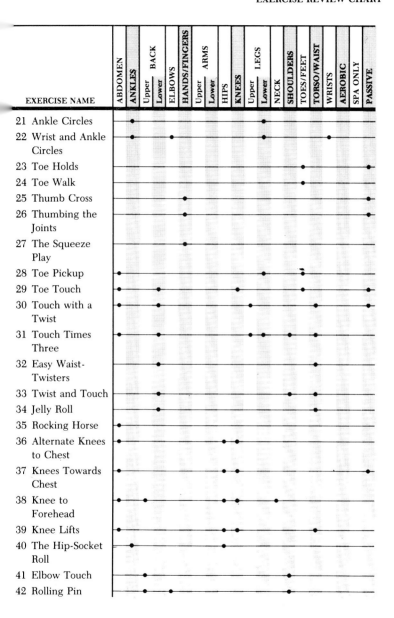

EXERCISE NAME	ABDOMEN	ANKLES	BACK Upper	BACK Lower	ELBOWS	HANDS/FINGERS	ARMS Upper	ARMS Lower	HIPS	KNEES	LEGS Upper	LEGS Lower	NECK	SHOULDERS	TOES/FEET	TORSO/WAIST	WRISTS	AEROBIC	SPA ONLY	PASSIVE
21 Ankle Circles		•										•								
22 Wrist and Ankle Circles		•			•							•					•			
23 Toe Holds															•					•
24 Toe Walk															•					
25 Thumb Cross						•														
26 Thumbing the Joints						•														
27 The Squeeze Play						•														
28 Toe Pickup	•									•					•					
29 Toe Touch	•			•						•	•									•
30 Touch with a Twist	•			•						•	•									•
31 Touch Times Three	•			•						•	•			•		•				
32 Easy Waist-Twisters				•												•				
33 Twist and Touch				•										•		•				
34 Jelly Roll	•																			
35 Rocking Horse	•																			
36 Alternate Knees to Chest	•								•											
37 Knees Towards Chest	•								•	•								•		•
38 Knee to Forehead	•	•							•	•	•									
39 Knee Lifts	•								•	•										
40 The Hip-Socket Roll		•							•											
41 Elbow Touch			•																	
42 Rolling Pin			•		•									•						•

145

EXERCISE REVIEW CHART

EXERCISE NAME	ABDOMEN	ANKLES	Upper BACK	Lower BACK	ELBOWS	HANDS/FINGERS	Upper ARMS	Lower ARMS	HIPS	KNEES	Upper LEGS	Lower LEGS	NECK	SHOULDERS	TOES/FEET	TORSO/WAIST	WRISTS	AEROBIC	SPA ONLY	PASSIVE
43 Front Kick	●								●											●
44 Leg Lifts and Swings	●								●	●										
45 Kick Lift	●								●	●										
46 Up and Out	●								●											
47 Easy 8s	●								●											
48 Lazy 8s	●								●											
49 8s the Hard Way	●								●											
50 Lazy 8s the Hard Way	●								●											
51 Ankle Lifts	●								●						●					
52 The Winner							●							●						●
53 Horizontal Wrist Circles						●	●							●						●
54 Vertical Wrist Circles			●											●		●				●
55 Shoulder Touch					●															
56 Assisted Rotating Palms					●															
57 Finger Spread						●														
58 Finger Backbends						●											●			
59 Assisted Finger Curls						●														●
60 Thumb Circles						●														●
61 Top-Bends						●														●
62 Thumb Up and Over						●														●
63 Assisted Leg Lift	●								●											●
64 Foot Slide									●	●										●
65 Assisted Push and Pull									●											●

EXERCISE NAME	ABDOMEN	ANKLES	Upper BACK	Lower BACK	ELBOWS	HANDS/FINGERS	Upper ARMS	Lower ARMS	HIPS	KNEES	Upper LEGS	Lower LEGS	NECK	SHOULDERS	TOES/FEET	TORSO/WAIST	WRISTS	AEROBIC	SPA ONLY	PASSIVE
66 One Foot Helps the Other		●																		●
67 Toe Bends		●													●					●
68 Toe Bends by Hand															●					●
69 Foot-Waving by Hand		●													●					●
70 Foot Circles by Hand		●													●					●
71 Waist Press							●	●	●											
72 Tummy Flatteners	●															●				
73 Forehead Flattener							●	●	●				●							
74 Chin Thrust													●							
75 Elbow to Elbow							●		●											
76 Prayer Position							●		●											
77 Extended Prayer Position							●		●											
78 Fist-over-Fist Press							●		●											
79 Finger Press							●	●	●											
80 Thigh Press							●		●											
81 Knee/Palm Press	●						●	●	●		●									●
82 Criss-Crossed Wrists							●	●	●		●									
83 Criss-Crossed Forearms							●	●			●									
84 Tug-of-War							●		●		●									
85 Toe Tug-of-War	●										●		●		●					
86 Bottle Bounce							●	●	●											
87 Bottle Press							●	●	●											

147

EXERCISE REVIEW CHART

EXERCISE NAME	ABDOMEN	ANKLES	BACK Upper	BACK Lower	ELBOWS	HANDS/FINGERS	ARMS Upper	ARMS Lower	HIPS	KNEES	LEGS Upper	LEGS Lower	NECK	SHOULDERS	TOES/FEET	TORSO/WAIST	WRISTS	AEROBIC	SPA ONLY	PASSIVE
88 Foot Press										●	●				●					
89 Reach for the Gold					●	●								●		●		●		
90 Crossovers	●						●		●	●				●				●		
91 Swing Your Elbows				●	●									●				●		
92 Breaststroke Triangle					●		●							●				●		
93 Foot Drag	●														●			●		
94 Tricycle	●	●							●	●								●		
95 Arm and Leg Co-ordination		●			●		●	●	●	●				●				●		
96 Flutter Kick	●																		●	
97 Great Big Circles		●												●		●			●	●
98 Ballet Bend				●										●		●	●	●		
99 Body Twists				●										●				●		
100 Crazy Legs	●								●	●								●		
101 Single-Leg Triangles	●								●	●								●		
102 Reverse Single-Leg Triangles	●								●	●								●		
103 Froggie Kick	●								●									●		
104 Reverse Froggie Kick	●						●		●									●		
105 Elementary Backstroke					●		●							●				●		
106 Elementary Backstroke with Kick	●				●		●	●	●	●				●				●		●
107 Hand Massage						●														
108 Elbow Massage					●	●	●													
109 Elbow-to-Shoulder Massage						●								●						

148

EXERCISE NAME	ABDOMEN	ANKLES	Upper BACK	Lower BACK	ELBOWS	HANDS/FINGERS	Upper ARMS	Lower ARMS	HIPS	KNEES	Upper LEGS	Lower LEGS	NECK	SHOULDERS	TOES/FEET	TORSO/WAIST	WRISTS	AEROBIC	SPA ONLY	PASSIVE
110 Finger Walking					●	●	●	●						●						
111 Upper-Leg Massage										●	●									
112 Lower-Leg Massage										●		●								
113 Full-Leg Massage	●									●	●									
114 Finger Jogging	●									●	●	●								
115 Foot Kneading															●					
116 Gentle Circles															●					
117 Foot-to-Foot Massage															●					

149

Index